4988296

B/Pic

PEMBERTON, J.
Will Pickles of
Wensleydale

WILL PICKLES
OF WENSLEYDALE

WILL PICKLES
OF WENSLEYDALE

The Life of a Country Doctor

BY
JOHN PEMBERTON

PUBLISHED BY
GEOFFREY BLES · LONDON
1970

Printed in Great Britain
by Cox & Wyman Ltd,
Fakenham

SBN: 7138 0279 0

Published by
GEOFFREY BLES LTD
52 Doughty Street, London, W.C.1.N. 2LZ
36–38 Clarence Street, Sydney, N.S.W. 2000
532 Little Collins Street, Melbourne, C.1
246 Queen Street, Brisbane
CML Building, King William Street, Adelaide, S.A. 5000
Lake Road, Northcote, Auckland
100 Lesmill Road, Don Mills, Ontario
P.O. Box 8879, Johannesburg
P.O. Box 834, Cape Town
P.O. Box 2800, Salisbury, Rhodesia

To My Wife

THIS WAS HIS PATH

This was his path . . . by farm and byre
A Northern road to tread;
The Ure in spate or under snow,
The skylark overhead.
Cloud shadows dark across the Dale,
By every Bridge and bend
The blowing daffodils of Spring,
The fell frosts of back-end.

Wind shakes the trees, year in year out,
Full-blown, December bare:
He knows each face and cottage door,
Each hearth and narrow stair;
The rain's song and the river's song,
The living and the dead
And all the troubles and the pains,
He cured and comforted.

And though with fame he travelled far,
Saw flying fish and foam
And cities half the world away
Always his heart turned home
To curlews crying, heather hills,
A rainbow on the falls . . .
His own house with its high beech hedge
And little grey stone walls.

Early and late, the seasons through,
This was the path he chose,
A country doctor on his rounds . . .
And everybody knows
His voice, his smile, the way he walks,
His presence in the Vale;
They will remember evermore
His name in Wensleydale.

Joan Pomfret
September 1951

CONTENTS

References

References to Dr. Pickles's published works are numbered in the text and given in date order in Appendix 1. Other references are printed as footnotes.

ILLUSTRATIONS

IN TEXT

ACKNOWLEDGEMENTS

I am grateful to Joan Pomfret for permission to publish "This was his path" and to the following for allowing me to publish charts, photographs and extracts:

John Wright & Sons Ltd., The Lancet, The British Medical Journal, The Practitioner, Medical News, The Guardian, The Birmingham Post and Mail, The Yorkshire Post, C. H. Wood (Bradford) Ltd., The Nuffield Foundation, George W. Hare, Dr. Stuart Carne and R. B. Fawcett.

INTRODUCTION

THIS BOOK GREW out of a series of locums I did for Will Pickles when his partners went away for their summer holidays.

Knowing of his work on epidemiology in country practice, I asked him when we first met in 1949 if I could visit him and see his charts of epidemics of infectious disease. He suggested that I might like to combine this with a fortnight's locum and I readily accepted the invitation. In writing to confirm the arrangements he added a post-script:

"His feet are clay although his face is brass
And this you will discover before the fortnight pass."

For the next ten years, with only one break, I spent part of my summer holiday doing this most enjoyable of locums. Every after-noon I would walk over from the George and Dragon to his house and we would discuss the day's visits over a cup of tea. Will would tell me about the past illnesses of the patients and their lives, and this would lead on to stories of an earlier generation in Wensleydale. Later on in the evening I would go back to his house, and the conversation would turn to his epidemiological work and the many friends he had made as a consequence of his journeys to America, Australia and South Africa. Sometimes he would talk about his father, Dr. John Pickles, and his childhood in Leeds. Whenever he was at a loss for a date or a name he would ask Gerty (Mrs. Pickles) to look it up, and Gerty unfailingly turned up the record from her notebooks.

Sometimes we met during the morning round, although usually

we went to opposite ends of the dale. I recall seeing him on one cold
autumnal morning walking across the market place at Askrigg. He
was hatless, and his unbuttoned mackintosh blew out behind him
in the strong wind. In one hand he clutched three or four bottles of
medicine, and with the other he waved to an old lady standing in a
doorway. Above his head the golden hands of the clock on the
church tower glinted on the brown stone as the sun appeared for a
moment, and then the rain started beating down again on the sets,
and the trees in the churchyard bent to the wind. Will Pickles was
part of the Yorkshire scene.

For more than fifty years he served his patients in Wensleydale
with skill and devotion, and although this earned him a special
place in the memories and affections of generations of dalesfolk, it
would not alone have ensured him a place in medical history. It is
because he also found time to make carefully recorded observations
on cases of infectious disease for more than a quarter of a century,
and found time to analyse and write about these in an interesting and
attractive way, that he is known far beyond Wensleydale and will
be remembered by future generations of doctors. His particular
contributions to medical knowledge are that he was one of the first
to identify and describe Bornholm disease in Great Britain, and by
his observations of the natural history of infectious hepatitis, then
called catarrhal jaundice, he was able to confirm accurately the long
incubation period first suggested by Booth and Okell. His description of Bornholm disease is so vivid and accurate that it has
become one of the classical descriptions of disease. He also described
and was the first to suggest the name "Farmer's Lung" for the
disabling condition brought about by repeated inhalation of the dust
from mouldy hay.

It is a remarkable fact that he did not start his epidemiological
inquiries until he was over forty, at a time when he might have
chosen to remain content to devote himself to his practice, his family
and the pleasant social life of the dale.

He developed a simple but useful method of charting all the new
cases of the infectious diseases which he saw. Each new case was
noted down in his pocket diary, even in the hectic days of an
influenza epidemic, with the name, place and date of onset, and the

information was transferred by Gerty to a time chart on which the villages that made up the practice were kept separate. About once a fortnight Gerty would bring the charts up to date from the pocket diary, but during epidemics they were done daily. Each disease had its own coloured symbol (see chart, facing p. 114). Over the first twenty years of his observations 6,808 cases of infectious disease were recorded, made up as follows:

Diarrhoea and vomiting	1,562	German measles	177
Influenza	1,320	Hepatitis	149
Febrile catarrh	968	Scarlet fever	125
Measles	569	Glandular fever	62
Tonsillitis	479	Lobar pneumonia	50
Chicken-pox	411	Bornholm disease	39
Whooping-cough	390	Diphtheria	12
Mumps	278	Anterior poliomyelitis	4
Zoster	213	Total	6,808

From these charts and his intimate knowledge of the lives of his patients, Will was often able to trace the source and spread of epidemics in the dale. He was always on the look-out for what he called "the short and only possible contact". A chance meeting in a pub, at a wedding or a funeral, enabled him to establish accurately the incubation period of an infectious disease and sometimes the period of infectiousness. It might require patient and tactful questioning to uncover some unsuspected contact, perhaps a secret love affair, and thus provide the key to a new outbreak in a village. But this Will was often able to do.

The chart reproduced facing page 114 shows, for example, how three crops of cases of measles occurred in the village of West Witton at intervals of about two weeks following a single initial case and how it then passed to Thoralby. It also shows how at the same time West Witton remained free from influenza for three months, although there was quite an epidemic occurring in the other villages. It is doubtful whether a village would escape for so long today, now that communication between villages by private car and motor cycle has increased so much. It is partly because these contacts were infrequent when Will was studying his epidemics that he was so often able to trace the spread of an infectious disease.

A Lancet reviewer of his Milroy lectures in 1942 epitomised the scene:

"These lectures breathe the spirit of the countryside and it is easy to visualise with the author the cheerful high spirited busloads of country folk exchanging jokes and germs as they make their pilgrimages from the Wensleydale villages to market or to cinema in country towns. One can imagine that Pickles knows them all, their families, their stock, their merits and their human failings".

Will often referred to the village summer outing and the Christmas visit to Leeds as "the replenishers of the bacterial flora of the dale".

Once started on his epidemiological enquiries he found them of absorbing interest, and when he described his work to the Epidemiological Section of the Royal Society of Medicine in 1935 he said:[6]

"To assess it at its lowest value, this has proved to me a most interesting hobby, something to turn the face from the clod and to add interest to the daily round, which, instead of being monotonous, becomes full of delightfully exciting incidents".

He often referred in his writings to this aspect of his work and in 1950 wrote:[19]

"Sir Thomas Browne in his *Religio Medici* writes: 'I feel it not in me those sordid and unchristian desires of my profession; I do not secretly implore and wish for plagues', but", Will continued, "one is human and the presence of a little infectious disease is not without its thrill."

On another occasion he said about his epidemiological enquiries:

"I get very enthusiastic and I think of very little else. 'Farmers' Lung' absolutely seized me. What a joy it was to feel you were on to something that isn't very well known."

He often said, "I have had a lot of luck in life", and he was perhaps fortunate in that first Dr. Alison Glover of the Ministry of Health

took an interest in his work in the early 1930s, and that later Professor
Major Greenwood recognised its importance and encouraged him
to write a book about it. These contacts only came because he was
ready to seek advice and to keep himself up-to-date by attending courses and meetings in London. The book he finally
wrote, *Epidemiology in Country Practice*,[10] a slender volume of
112 pages, was first published in 1939 and has become a medical
classic.

It is rare for a general practitioner to become famous in the field
of medicine. Perhaps this is because it is difficult for a G.P. to
concentrate on a single problem when continually confronted with
the whole spectrum of disease at any time of the day or night.

Will Pickles follows in the line of only a handful of G.Ps. who
have achieved fame in British medicine; his predecessors are Edward
Jenner who discovered the effectiveness of vaccination with cow-pox
against small-pox, William Budd who discovered the mode of
transmission of typhoid fever and James Mackenzie who invented a
method of recording the pulse waves and thereby greatly improved
the accuracy of diagnosis and prognosis in heart disease. Will Pickles
showed once again that the general practitioner has unique opportunities for making observations on disease which are denied to other
medical men, and in his book he quotes William Budd on this
point:

> "Having been born and brought up in the village, I was personally
> acquainted with every inhabitant of it; and being, as a medical
> practitioner, in almost exclusive possession of the field, nearly every
> one who fell ill, not only in the village itself, but over a large area
> round it came immediately under my care.
>
> "For tracing the part of personal intercourse in the propagation
> of disease, better outlook could not possibly be had."*

Apart from his original contributions to medical knowledge,
Will's great service has been to demonstrate to general practitioners
throughout the world that it is possible for the G.P. to make original
and valuable observations on disease providing he has the patience
and industry. He advised all young doctors and medical students to

* William Budd (1811–80), *Typhoid fever, its nature, mode of spreading and prevention*

read the life of Mackenzie.* "It shows," he wrote, "how Mackenzie began to take notes of all his patients and then decided to narrow it down to those whose signs and symptoms were connected with the heart and that was where general practice came in. There was continuity. He was waiting to see what would happen to men, women and children who showed these symptoms and he was able to wait as we in general practice are able to wait."

Since Will's epidemiological work was completed a revitalisation of general practice in Great Britain has begun. The creation of the College of General Practitioners in 1953, which became the Royal College of General Practitioners in 1967, has been largely responsible for this. It is impossible to assess fully the contribution that Will's work made to the creation of the College, and to the many research projects which have since been carried out in general practice following this. The fact that he was elected its first president suggests that in the eyes of his fellow G.Ps. he had played a great part.

Will Pickles was one of the minority of general practitioners who welcomed the introduction of the National Health Service and appreciated the new opportunities that it would bring to G.Ps. "I am sad that so little has been said lately on group practice in the new Health Service," he wrote in 1948. "In the opinion of many there was fresh hope for the efficiency of general practice in the suggestion that doctors should work, not as detached individuals, but in groups – and if any contemplation of research is present, work in groups is of the highest importance." He went on to suggest various research problems for doctors working in Health Centres. He also indicated the necessity for the general practitioner to form a close liaison with the director of a laboratory and with the local Medical Officer of Health. Twenty years later these developments were just getting under way.

It was not uncommon, until a few years ago, for general practitioners to be appointed part-time Medical Officers of Health for remote rural districts. Will held such an appointment for the Aysgarth rural district for many years, and this may have been one of the reasons why he turned his attention to the epidemiology of

* R. McNair Wilson, *The Beloved Physician: Sir James Mackenzie*. John Murray, 1926

infectious disease. On several occasions the words "Medical Officer of Health, Aysgarth Rural District" appear after his name as author of an article, and one feels he was proud to hold this modest position in the public health service.

In writing this book I have had the unique advantage of being allowed to read and to quote from much of Will's own unpublished autobiographical writings, and for this I am deeply grateful. Over a period of nineteen years I had many conversations with him and the reader will readily discern how much the book owes to its subject. I have tried to place his work in the perspective of his life as a country doctor.

What sort of man emerges? I think that the overwhelming impression that Will Pickles made upon his friends was one of warmth of character and friendly geniality. His welcoming words to patient or friend alike and uttered with a beaming smile, "Now old man, come in," made the visitor feel that Will was truly pleased to see him.

He suffered fools courteously if not gladly, and a very old lady in one of the villages recalled how "he used to bow a lot" when he first came to practice in Wensleydale. His punctuality was part of the same trait. This and his habit of writing everything down no doubt helped him to get through his work efficiently as well as to carry out his epidemiological inquiries. There was also a tough streak in his character. He once said, "I do things because I like doing them and I never did like doing things from a sense of duty".

Some doctors treat their patients as opponents, some as malingerers, some are afraid of them and some treat them as though they are feeble-minded. Will treated all his patients, rich and poor, shy or demanding, as human beings.

I never heard him disparage a patient. One day a young locum was reporting on his round to Will, and as he came to each name, it seemed that every patient was either exaggerating his symptoms, was too stupid to carry out the treatment advised, or was obviously malingering. The locum seemed to have reprimanded them all. Finally, at the end of the recital, Will, losing his customary urbanity, angrily remarked: "You *can't* treat these people like that. I've known them for a lifetime – they're *good* people."

In country districts where there may be no choice of doctor, the contentment or misery of a lot of people may depend on the character of the local doctor. If he is kind and conscientious, as so many are, he can bring ease of mind to many sick people. If he is lazy, selfish and indifferent he may only add to their suffering.

In carrying out his investigations, Will found the dales folk helpful and interested. Even when he undertook to investigate the frequency of cousin marriages for a national enquiry into heredity disease he found that they were willing to give information on this highly personal matter.

Over the years he received much assistance and support from Gerty in his work, which he frequently acknowledged. Soon after their marriage she had got into the habit of jotting down the daily events which seemed important to her on the left-hand page of her grocery book. Later, as the horizon broadened, not only did she maintain the epidemiological charts with meticulous care, but also kept a record of their journeys together. The details were accurately recorded and whenever they met someone for the first time Gerty seems to have ascertained his initials, the proper spelling of his surname and his exact occupation. The notebooks were not just dry lists of names and meetings, however. They contain passages which reveal a delicate sensitivity to people and places.

I had the privilege of reading these private records and of quoting from them.

Aysgarth became something of a medical Mecca in the 1950s. Doctors from all over the world with an interest in epidemiology would call at this rather inaccessible little village in the North Riding of Yorkshire in order to meet Will and see the district in which he did his work. Perhaps I cannot do better in setting the scene of his life than to quote the passage which he sometimes used to introduce his lectures:

"I recall a particularly lovely evening in early summer, when I climbed alone to the summit of one of our noble hills. The sun was setting and it lit up the grim pile of an ancient castle, once the prison of history's unhappiest queen, our little lake seemed to lie at my feet and one by one I made out most of our grey villages with their thin pall of smoke. And as I watched the evening train creeping up the valley with its pauses at our three stations, a quaint thought came into my head and it was that there was hardly a man, woman or child in all those villages of whom I did not know the Christian name and with whom I was not on terms of intimate friendship. My wife and I say that we know most of the dogs and, indeed, some of the cats."

Will Pickles enjoyed almost every minute of his professional life. He could have gone to the Ministry of Health as an epidemiologist in 1931, but as he himself said of country doctors:

"They tend to remain in one practice and to become part of their district. There is something in country practice – I believe it is the deep bonds of friendship between doctor and patient – that breeds content, and it would be unthinkable in most of us to change our habitat . . . I made my decision in favour of a country practice with my eyes open knowing full well that the remuneration would never compare with that of my town colleagues, but I would not have spent my life elsewhere for all the wealth of the Indies."

I

CHILDHOOD

WILLIAM NORMAN PICKLES was born on 6th March, 1885, in Camp Road, Leeds. His mother, Lucy, was attended in her confinement by her husband, Dr. John Jagger Pickles, and this was the second of the six sons she was to bear. All were destined to enter the medical profession, although by the time Charles, the youngest, went to medical school, the family urge to doctoring had perhaps weakened a little. He alone of the six brothers failed to qualify.

Will's ancestors, with the exception of a Scottish grandmother on the maternal side, were Yorkshiremen and women, and the commonly recognised qualities of this race – kindliness, mental toughness and a love of the ribald jest – were later to develop in him to the full.

On the paternal side it was his grandfather, Philip Pickles, who initiated the family interest in healing for he, in addition to keeping the post office in the village of Shelf, near Bradford, was the local pharmacist and tooth extractor. He also advised on the diagnosis and treatment of common ailments when called upon, for doctors in those days were scarce, and a luxury – or a charity – for the poor. Will, at the age of four, was taken to view the body of Philip Pickles as he lay in his coffin, but the event made little impression upon him.

Will's father, John Pickles, went to Hipperholme Grammar School where he did well. When he left school he went to work for a few months in a leading chemist's shop in Leeds, a valuable training in dispensing, before entering Leeds Medical School.

Several of Will's mother's relatives were doctors. One of them, her uncle Thomas Dobson, was a general practitioner in Leeds. He seems to have been a remarkable old man who lived to a great age, and Will's recollections of him bring vividly back the medical scene in the 1890s. When he retired the old men of Holbeck gave him a dinner and many nice things were said about him. In his speech he queried whether he was the person in question. He thought he could not be the man referred to as "all his days were spent in mixing spirits and many of his nights with other men's wives." In his old age he had a strangulated hernia which was operated on by a surgeon at the Leeds Infirmary known as "Gaffer" Brown who drove a four-wheel dogcart drawn by a pair of bays and whose face was brick-red from exposure to the weather, but he was beautifully turned out with his spotless white muffler. Unfortunately Dr. Dobson developed a haemorrhage a few days later and a Dr. Woodcock was called in. Not knowing quite what to do he took out his bicycle and sped off to "Gaffer" Brown's house in Woodhouse Lane, but no response was given to his urgent ringing of the bell. Finally he left and contacted the young Moynihan, who fetched out his own bicycle and cycled with Dr. Woodcock to Holbeck, where he dealt with the haemorrhage. Brown was much upset and explained that he had never heard the bell. He was a great entertainer and that night he had had Conan Doyle staying with him.

Will's mother, Lucy Dobson, was the daughter of a marriage which had foundered and Lucy, with her sister Annie, was brought up in an uncle's home. For some time she had obtained posts as a governess but later started a dame school with her sister. This modest enterprise was subsequently ruined by an outbreak of scarlet fever in which several of the children died.

When Will was born, his father, John Pickles was thirty-five and his mother a year younger. The first twenty-five years of his life were spent in Camp Road which was then a dreary, shabby, genteel neighbourhood in the centre of Leeds. Today it is a slum undergoing demolition.

When he was two, the family moved to a larger house, across the road which had seven bedrooms and large gloomy attics that the little boy was afraid to enter. The family income at that time (1887) was approximately eight hundred pounds a year, and they were able to employ a nanny, a cook and a housemaid. Each of the domestics was paid about eighteen pounds a year, and each received a new apron and half a crown at Christmas. Sarah, the nanny, tried to obtain good behaviour from her charges by warning them of what would happen to them at the Last Trump if they were disobedient. This so impressed itself on William's mind that an itinerant trumpeter who chanced to play before the house one night filled him with terror, as he was convinced that the Day of Judgement had come.

Sunday was a miserable day. The children were not allowed to bicycle or even to draw or paint. In consequence, they would try and persuade their parents to take them to Harewood Church instead of their local place of worship, as this would at least ensure an interesting walk in the country. William's father, Dr. John Pickles, although not blessed with deep religious conviction, was a great church-goer. The sermons, long and tedious to Will, were the only part his father enjoyed. The doctor would contrive to arrive just before the sermon, giving the impression that he had been detained by a sudden call from a patient.

At the age of four, Will was sent to a little school run by his aunt and was sadly disillusioned to discover how sternly a dearly loved relation could behave in the classroom, even to her own kin. After two years there, he went to school at the Quaker Meeting House in Woodhouse Lane, where he stayed until his education began in earnest at Leeds Grammar School which he entered at the age of nine.

At about this time he decided he would like to become a parson, and that he would continue his drawing and painting, to which he was very much attached, as side lines. Once every two years the whole family went to Whitby or Morecambe for a fortnight's holiday, and Will would spend hours sketching the cliffs and boats or Whitby Abbey. At these times, a locum would be appointed to look after the practice and an aunt would move in to look after the locum. Sarah, the nanny accompanied the family to the seaside. As the children grew up, Sarah gradually exchanged the duties of nanny for cook. Like so many of her almost extinct class, she remained with the family long after the boys had grown up and gone out into the world. Altogether she was with the Pickles for sixty years, and only left in the end when an unexpected legacy enabled her to spend her last days in the comparative ease of a nursing-home. On alternate years Dr. and Mrs. Pickles would go farther afield and visit Norway and Switzerland, and at these times the older boys would take an old bell-tent and go and camp on a farm near their grandmother's in the country north of the city, and later in Wensleydale.

As the family enlarged, so the occasions for family festivals increased. Birthdays and Christmas were invariably celebrated with all the domestic rituals. The Christmas Eve dinner-party was a great occasion. Some two dozen of them would sit down to the feast; eight Pickles, ten Dobsons, with perhaps two or three wives and fiancées and Dr. Gordon Sharpe, a Scottish neighbour.

There was roast turkey, a roast goose, a couple of boiled fowls, roast ham and always a jugged hare, all beautifully served with roast potatoes, mashed potatoes and potatoes in their jackets, brussel sprouts and cauliflowers, followed by plum pudding, mince pies and trifles and a large cheese. The church choir came and sang carols after dinner and a band played cheerful tunes.

On New Year's Eve the Pickles went to the Dobsons and were similarly entertained.

Discipline in the home was maintained mainly by the strict and upright character of Lucy Pickles, whose standards, derived from her Quaker ancestry, were high and unwavering. She was an advocate for old age pensions, to stave off the dreaded workhouse, years before they were introduced, and she showed great sympathy for the problems of unmarried mothers at a time when condemnation was the general attitude. She was very religious and was the dominating influence in the household. An occasional beating from his father might be required to emphasise a point of discipline and these were resented for years by Will, who later felt that they had done little good. Although somewhat severe with his sons, John Pickles was a sociable man, and every Thursday evening the Pickles held open house for medical colleagues, clerics and other friends. They would enjoy supper, drinks and cigars, and afterwards in the drawing-room Will, who had a good ear and a sweet voice, might be asked to sing a ballad or a solo from an anthem before the company settled down to whist.

John Pickles had been one of the most distinguished students of his year at the Leeds General Infirmary, obtaining several medals and prizes. After qualification, he had become House Physician to the great Dr. Clifford Albutt, who had christened him "the *vis à tergo*" and he later became Resident Medical Officer at the Infirmary. He maintained a close association with his alma mater. He would visit his patients when they were admitted to hospital, and took great pains to get to know every new member of the hospital staff. Such was his attachment to Clifford Albutt, that tears would come into his eyes when his old chief spoke to him, and he named his third son after him.

He had entered general practice by putting up his plate in Camp Road, and on account of his great energy he soon attained a considerable reputation for his skill, particularly in midwifery, and as a result he was called to confinements in all parts of Leeds. Often he would first see the expectant mother when she was in labour as there was little in the way of antenatal care in those days.

He had few interests outside his professional work and in that he possessed an unusual curiosity. Medicine at the end of the nineteenth century was still very much more of an "art" than a science. "I can always bluff them," he would say, referring to the persistent type of patient. "If they ask me what's wrong with them, I say to them, 'that's my business. Do as I tell you and take your medicine and you'll get better'." Although he may have bluffed his patients, he never bluffed himself, and when they died, as they quite often did, he would, if he were uncertain of the cause of death, persuade the relatives to allow him to carry out a post-mortem examination in the home. Later on, Will would assist him in these sombre searches after the truth.

At that time, apart from surgical procedures, themselves hazardous because of the danger of sepsis, there were few specific remedies and none with the miraculous curative qualities, for example, of penicillin. Mercury was of proven value for syphilis, digitalis for cardiac dropsy, and iron for chlorosis. If these were not appropriate, the patient could always be given a purgative or bromide, or, for those in pain, laudanum. For confinements, the family doctor had three aids: a drug, ergot, misused to hasten delivery, obstetric forceps, often misused for the same purpose and chloroform to render the suffering woman unconscious of all the efforts, good or bad, intended to assist her. To the intelligent young doctor not content with tradition and empiricism, the relatively new studies of pathology and bacteriology which were being rapidly developed by the use of the microscope and by post-mortem examinations, promised to provide a more rational and satisfactory basis for diagnosis and treatment.

John Pickles, like most general practitioners of those days, undertook a great deal of midwifery, and Will's earliest memories include that of a conversation repeated over and over again, the urgent words conveyed to his father's bedside by the night speaking tube:

"Doctor! Doctor! The child's coming," and his father's weary reply:

"All right, all right; I'm coming as quickly as ever I can."

John Pickles' midwifery record book was found after his death to contain the names of no less than 2,700 mothers whom he had attended in childbirth.

At night it was rarely possible to knock up the driver of the hired "growler" which the doctor used as a conveyance in the day-time to go on his rounds. The visits had often to be made on foot, through the dismal, ill-lit streets of Leeds, many of them not even paved. One night, when he had managed to hire a hansom to go to a woman in labour, he found when he at last came out into the street again that it was pouring with rain and the cab had vanished. He guessed what had happened and walked round to a near-by inn where he found the cabby much the worse for drink. He bundled him into his own cab and himself mounted to the driver's seat and drove home. On such occasions he used to say to his family: "When I reach a thousand a year, I'll buy a horse and carriage of my own"; but he never did.

He always wore a frock coat and well-brushed top hat until he acquired a bicycle on which to do his rounds. He then changed over to knickerbockers and a tweed coat, but still on occasions wore his frock coat over the knickerbockers for special visits.

When Will entered Leeds Grammar School, John Henry Dudly Matthews was headmaster. He was a classical scholar and a clergyman, and science teaching, as was usual then, occupied a very humble place in the curriculum. Perhaps this was the reason why Will from an early age loved Greek above all subjects. This attitude was not appreciated by his schoolfellows, one of whom, on hearing Will's confession of his predilection, insisted with some show of violence that what he really meant was that he hated Greek least. He did indeed hate mathematics and did not at first seem to have any scientific inclination. Later on, however, he managed to learn the rudiments of chemistry, physics and mechanics.

At first, he did not take much part in organised games at school because he was afraid to stay behind after lessons were over as there was a school bully – a German boy – who tormented the small fry. Eventually Will was goaded on to fight one of the bully's lieutenants who also happened to be the headmaster's son, and having defeated this "jackal" he found that thereafter he was left in peace. He became fond of rugby and gained a place in the second fifteen. He also used to swim and to box with his Dobson cousins.

He did well in most subjects at school; he was never late and rarely punished. His cousin, Jo Dobson, on the other hand, was often late and was compelled to learn Greek verses as a punishment, so that in later life he could recite much of Homer by heart. At the age of eleven Will won a scholarship in the school which earned his family a remission of fees for the rest of his school days. He was top of the fifth form and entered the sixth form at the early age of fifteen.

Owing to the enlightened views of the headmaster, the sixth form boys were allowed to organise their own work to a large extent and spent much time in the well-stocked library which was regarded rather like a club. Will made full use of the library and read with enjoyment Dickens, Thackeray, Trollope and Jane Austen.

He enjoyed the debates of the school debating society but because of his shyness, he could not bring himself to speak in public. Indeed he did not overcome this feeling for nearly fifty years.

His early desire to become a man of religion with a part-time interest in art soon faded in the face of the family example. He admired his father deeply, and the way he responded to the urgent calls of the sick. His elder brother Philip had already decided to study medicine, his mother was ambitious and pressed them on, so the decision to become a doctor was natural, almost inevitable.

He had no difficulty in qualifying for entrance to university by passing the London matriculation examination in which he was placed in the first division. He also obtained a Leeds

Infirmary scholarship which covered the fees for the last two years of the course.

Thus Will's childhood, on the whole happy and successful, came to an end. It had been passed in the famous years of a dying century; Gladstone had waged his unsuccessful struggle for Irish Home Rule; the Diamond Jubilee of Queen Victoria had been celebrated by a prosperous and complacent nation, and a few years later, her death mourned as a national disaster. The Boer war had been bitterly fought and won. To the schoolboy, these events were probably less real than his love of Greek, his fear of the German bully or the excitement of a game of rugby.

His childhood came to an end as the new century was beginning. The medicine of the brougham and galenicals was fading away into the past. The medicine of the motor-car, salvarsan, insulin, sulphonamides and the anti-biotics was on its way. Will entered the medical school of the Yorkshire College in the Easter term of 1902, just after his seventeenth birthday.

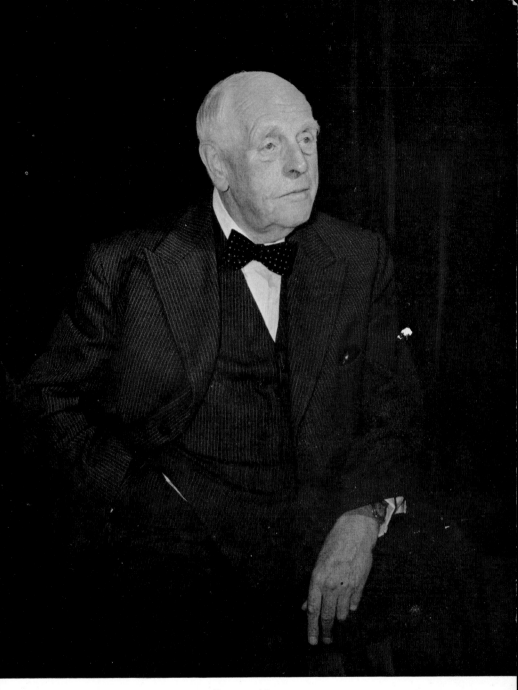

Dr. William Pickles in 1956

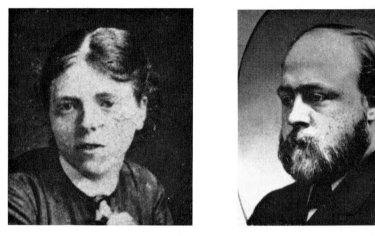

Will's parents; Lucy (1852–1917) and Dr. John (1851–1925)

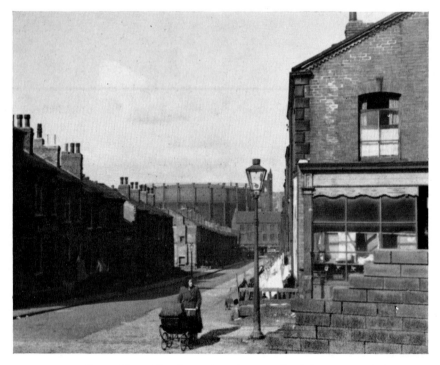

From Camp Road, Leeds, where Will's father practised

2

MEDICAL STUDENT

IN THOSE DAYS there was less difficulty than today in entering a medical school providing that the candidate had matriculated and his parents could afford the fees. One of the results of selection today, based on a high level of academic performance and the system of local education authority grants dependent upon continued success, is the virtual disappearance of the "perpetual student" from our medical schools. To the older generation of doctors he was a colourful character who had often taken time off from his studies to develop a sideline of interest to him, and who, because he was quite willing to spend two years over what most men hurried through in one, was able to act as a guardian of tradition and link between the old and the new.

When Will entered the medical school of the Yorkshire College which was later to become part of the University of Leeds, there was a student of eleven years standing who, by being able to devote sufficient time to the game, had been captain of the Yorkshire rugby team for several years. The times were leisurely, society more stable. If your parents could afford a college education for you, you could have it, no matter if it did take rather longer than usual to acquire a degree. The territory of "scholars and gentlemen" was still well preserved and there were only a few narrow gateways through which the brilliant poor boy might squeeze by means of scholarships. The "eleven plus" examination and the breaking down of the social fences which surrounded the professions was a generation ahead.

Will continued to live at his parents' house. He returned home to lunch and at the weekends went walking or cycling with his brothers or cousins. Indeed, he did not finally leave the parental home until he was twenty-five, a circumstance that he afterwards regretted. One of the results of these close family ties was that he did not become immersed in student activities. He did however join the Student Christian Movement. In spite of a desire for a settled faith by which to live, final conviction never came and even before he became a doctor he had, while accepting the Christian ethic, adopted the agnostic position which was to be his attitude to religion throughout his life.

He was not selected for students' committees or the students' representative council, probably because of a natural distaste for expressing himself in public. He often went with his brothers and cousins to private subscription dances and later on in his career, if he arrived late because of dispensing or hospital work, his girl cousins had no difficulty in getting his programme filled up before he arrived.

His failure to pass his First M.B. at the first attempt suggests that after leaving school work no longer occupied the whole, or even a great deal of his attention. His thoughts were perhaps deflected by the subscription dances and by the entrancing maidens who glided towards him in the lancers or clung to him during the waltzes. One particular attachment to a pretty student nurse endured for several years, but in those days marriage as a student was unthinkable. There were no government grants and any additional cost would have to be borne by one's parents.

In his third year he won the anatomy prize and passed the examination that allowed him to proceed to his clinical studies in the Leeds General Infirmary.

There was very little systematic instruction for medical students in the hospital wards at the beginning of the century. The student, in "walking the wards", was expected to observe the methods of the "Olympians" when they made their weekly rounds in frock coats, and by imitation and practice, combined with judicious reading, gradually to acquire the Art of Medicine. At that time, the scientific knowledge underlying medicine was meagre, successful diagnosis depended more upon long experience than exact knowledge, and treatment was based largely upon tradition and authority. Departments of pathology were in their infancy; there were no departments of biochemistry and the use of X-Rays in diagnosis was undreamed of. Once the chief had examined the patient, a diagnosis had to be made and treatment prescribed. There was no possibility of suspending judgement or withholding treatment until the results of special investigations were available – there were none. Skilfully employed experience and a bold empiricism compounded with bluff and bedside manner, characterised many of the famous doctors of the day.

Will was Lord Moynihan's dresser for six months, and during this time was taught but twice by that brilliant and egotistical Irish surgeon. So vividly did Moynihan teach, however, that his pupil never forgot his views on the two subjects on which he did expound – stone in the bladder and thyroid disease. As a surgical dresser Will started at 7.30 in the morning carbolising wounds, washing out stomachs and dressing wounds, many of which were septic. Other duties included the catheterisation of coal miners whose backs had been broken by a fall of rock, the shaving with a cut-throat razor of patients for hernia operations, the extraction of teeth, the suture of wounds and the delicate operation of circumcision. These latter operations were not always performed with the nicety they deserved and it is said that on one occasion when a young resident doctor was making rather heavy weather of the procedure, the anaesthetist was heard to mutter: "There's a divinity that shapes our ends, rough-hew them how we will."

Many of the ward sisters ruled their wards with a rod of iron. They had to, to get the work done, because they had nothing like the number of nurses available today. The students were often frightened of them too. On one occasion when Will was having a friendly talk with a patient the sister came up and said in a loud voice "Mr. Pickles, don't you think it's time you stopped gossiping with this patient?"

Will was much influenced by Moynihan, who took a great interest in him. Once, at a medical dinner, Will's father said to Moynihan: "I expect you know my boy," to which the surgeon replied: "I look upon him as *my* boy." Years later, when Pickles began to report his epidemiological researches in the medical journals, Moynihan would always send a line with encouraging comments. On one occasion he wrote: "What you are doing is all to the good of British medicine." This letter was a great encouragement to Will.

Will was also medical clerk to Dr. Alfred Barrs, a witty and caustic physician. He would tell his clerks: "If a powerful drug is not doing good, it is probably doing harm." On one occasion some words he used left a deep and lasting impression on the young student's mind: "It is you general practitioners who should be the pioneers in medicine. You see patients in the beginning of their illnesses and can follow them through to the end."

The obstetric clerkship in the medical course provided Will with his first opportunity to observe at first hand the mean and sordid conditions under which so many people in Leeds were born and lived. Instruction in obstetrics was indifferent, and no one bothered to find out whether Will had even seen a baby born before he delivered his first. As it happened, when he arrived he found to his great relief that the child had already been born. Later on he became more effective. He learned to spread out the brown paper on the iron bedstead which had been trundled into the stone-floored kitchen. He learned to calm the frightened woman who paced about in her day clothes and who from time to time gripped the back of the kitchen chair as the pains of labour recurred with increasing frequency and severity. At first impatient with the old handy-women with their morbid prognostications and filthy appearance who came in to help on these occasions, Will came ultimately to tolerate and even respect them for the real comfort and practical help they gave in the dismal watches of the night. When the labour was obstructed or delayed, he would send a messenger to the hospital to ask the Resident Obstetric Officer to come quickly. This calm and superior being would then apply the forceps while Will administered chloroform. Later on, he became a skilful obstetrician himself, and would sometimes help his father in a difficult case.

Most medical students find that the study of sick men and women is of such absorbing interest that they have little time or even desire to become interested in literature, politics or art, although there are of course some notable exceptions. Will had developed a love of good writing before he started on his medical career and he continued to find time to read the works of the nineteenth century masters. On one occasion he combined his literary and medical knowledge in a paper on drug addiction which he read before the University Medical Society and illustrated by reference to the lake poets. His boyhood delight in drawing and painting was, however, never resumed.

When he was twenty he asked his father for permission to smoke, but was told to wait until he was twenty-one, and he did not take any alcohol until he was twenty-two. Even then he only drank beer except on those rare occasions which called for celebration with a ten shilling bottle of champagne.

Although not given to the rags and escapades usually enjoyed by medical students, he was once thrown out of a music hall with a group of fellow students who had attempted to shout down a certain quack and bone setter, "Dr." Bodie, who was giving a "faith healing" act. He escaped arrest on this occasion, but six of his fellows were not so lucky. The class subscribed to pay the fees of a lawyer and the magistrate dismissed the case. The medical school authorities, who were perhaps not entirely disinterested, turned a blind eye to the affair.

It was about this time that he became friendly with a fellow medical student, Dean Dunbar, who was later to be his partner at Aysgarth for twenty-two years and whose friendship proved to be one of the richest experiences of his life.

With four sons studying medicine at the same time, there was some financial hardship in the Pickles family, and to help the family in his final years Will dispensed for a general practitioner in the evenings. He worked from five to eight o'clock and was given tea and fifteen shillings a week. Quite often his employer would be called out on an urgent case in the middle of a surgery and he would then ask Will to see the rest of the patients. In this way, he became acquainted with some of the many problems that crop up in general practice. He began to learn how to distinguish trivial from serious disease from the way the patient told his story. He learned which patients must be thoroughly examined and which could be dismissed with a word of encouragement and a bottle of medicine. He gained experience in handling "difficult" patients and in temporising when he was by no means sure of the correct treatment. He also learned how book-keeping in general practice was done. After the evening surgery closed, he went home and studied until midnight, often taking a textbook to bed with him to try and absorb a few more pages before sleep overcame him.

The general practitioner, Dr. J. J. Anning, for whom Will dispensed at this time, was a remarkable man and took great pains to teach him clinical medicine. He later held a University lectureship. Among other talents he was skilled in penmanship. That Will was never guilty of the illegibility common among doctors is probably due to his example. Many years later, in an obituary notice for the British Medical Journal,[32] Will recorded his gratitude to Dr. Anning. "My position as dispenser meant much more than mere dispensary work and was akin to that of the medical apprentice of an earlier epoch. Many a time did he call me into his consulting room always giving me the impression that he would like my help and so giving me that confidence which means so much to young people. For this I have always been grateful to him."

It was not uncommon at that time for senior medical students to do locums for general practitioners who were sick or on holiday.

On one such occasion, Will had the use of a Victoria, a low, fast, doorless carriage, and when he was not busy he would drive up and down Headingley in the carriage imagining himself a fashionable physician. More often the principal would economise and send the dispenser and groom on holiday, and Will would spend hours looking perhaps for a bottle of *Tinct. Nux Vomica* on the stained and crowded shelves and pedalling round to visit the patients on a bicycle.

This practice of student locums occasionally led to the abuse of "covering". If a patient died while being attended by a student, another doctor would be asked to sign the medical certificate of the cause of death although he might never have seen the unfortunate patient before. Will thus became familiar with the makeshifts and contrivances of medical practice at that time as well as with some of the skills and qualities required.

The time came at last for him to take his final examinations. He first sat for the London M.B. in October 1908, and failed in both parts. He then lowered his sights and sat for the Licence of the Society of Apothecaries. This time he was more successful but was ploughed in clinical surgery. It was during this part of the examination that the examiner had shouted words which were never forgotten or forgiven: "What the hell did you say that for, Sir?".

In March 1909 he obtained his licence to qualify from the Society of Apothecaries and he lined up with the other successful candidates to receive his diploma in the ancient Apothecaries' Hall in Blackfriars. Within twenty-four hours of qualification, he had obtained a post as a locum tenens.

This was the first time he had lived away from home. He felt then that his experience of life had been restricted. Although there had been much to admire in the medical school there was much that was narrow. Like other provincial medical schools at that time, it was a world in itself, and the broader influence of the university which was only founded in 1904 had not yet permeated the medical school. As he entered the wider world he had to adapt himself to other households, to find himself work and balance his expenditure with his income; he had to make decisions and plan ahead. After working as a locum in various practices for some months, he felt he needed further training and took the opportunity of returning to the Leeds General Infirmary as Resident Obstetric Officer. Now, in his turn, he wore the mantle of a young god to those students sweating on the district when he came out to rescue them from their difficulties.

As was the custom in many teaching hospitals up to the Second World War, there was no salary attached to resident hospital appointments. In the six months of his tenure, he earned only fifteen pounds in fees from his chief for assisting at operations on private patients, and a few guineas for attending at inquests.

He was not satisfied with his L.S.A. qualification and continued to study for the London M.B. which his father had put forward years before as the proper objective for him, and after one or two unsuccessful attempts, he finally obtained this qualification in 1910.

Meantime Will's five brothers had either qualified in medicine or were preparing to become doctors.

His older brother, Philip, helped with the family expenses by dispensing and acting as a locum in the same way as Will. Unlike

Will, however, Philip had no intellectual curiosity; he was entirely absorbed by the human drama of medicine and did not acquire the habit of being able to detach himself from his patients' troubles which, so long as it never amounts to callousness, is an almost essential part of a doctor's training. Philip suffered with them. A few years after qualification, he was in H.M.S. *Russell* in the First World War when she was blown up in the Mediterranean. Although gassed with the fumes of burning cordite, he continued to attend the burned and injured seamen. He was rescued from the water after the *Russell* went down, but died a few hours later.

The next brother, Clifford, a year younger than Will, was his associate throughout the medical course. Each stimulated the other. Clifford approached his studies with a burning enthusiasm and would almost certainly have made his mark in the field of preventive medicine which he had selected for a career if he also had not died prematurely. He served in France, first as a combatant and later as a medical officer. He was never a happy man and suffered from trigeminal neuralgia and recurrent depression which led to his discharge from the army and his early death at the age of twenty-nine.

The fourth brother, Jack, went into practice at Leyburn, Wensleydale. He never married and never settled down happily in general practice. He acquired the reputation of being an eccentric and retired at the early age of forty-eight. Subsequently, when the Second World War broke out, he became a locum tenens for an absent colleague. He died from an obscure illness at the age of fifty-five.

Harold, the next brother, went into practice with his father in Leeds, and this enabled the older man in his later years to shed some of the heavy load of a city practice.

After their father retired, Harold found that the Leeds practice was too much to manage. He was a good business man and sold the practice for a substantial sum of money and then bought a smaller and waning practice in Kent intending to live less strenuously. Such was his personality however, that within three years the practice in Kent had grown to larger dimensions than the one he had given up. This he also sold together with the house he had built, at a considerable profit. He came to the North Riding again, and practised within twenty miles of Will. One stormy night in December 1944, Will answered the telephone to hear his brother's voice gasping that he had a severe pain in the chest. Ten days later at the age of fifty-three, he died in a Harrogate nursing home.

The sixth and last son, Charles, after failing to qualify as a doctor, wandered off first to South Africa and then to Canada. Later, he became a farmer, but was never successful and never married. He died at the age of thirty-eight.

Thus, of the six brothers, only Will survived into later life. Only two of the brothers married and only four children were born to this generation – a daughter to Will and two sons and a daughter to Harold.

3

EARLY YEARS IN GENERAL PRACTICE

DURING HIS APPOINTMENT as Resident Obstetric Officer, Will developed an ambition to become a gynaecologist and wanted to take additional appointments at the Leeds General Infirmary to gain experience. However, like many other young doctors who qualified in the days before junior hospital appointments were adequately paid or even paid at all, he could not afford to do this. In later life he never regretted his failure to specialise as this led in fact to his taking up the work he loved.

In July 1910 he obtained a locum in Moortown, a suburb of Leeds, and started his professional life in earnest. The doctor had gone away and Will was left to cope with the practice with only the advice of the servants who had been left behind in the large and gloomy house. Late on his first evening there was an emergency call; a woman was in labour. When Will arrived at the house the husband, a matter-of-fact Yorkshireman, was obviously put out at seeing this very young doctor on the doorstep instead of the principal. Having sized him up, he said to Will: "Well, young man, come on and let's see what you're made of."

Midwifery was one thing Will felt confident about. He gave an anaesthetic, put on the forceps and when it was all over the young mother said that if she had to go through it all again, she would have Will to do the job. He began to feel that he was a real doctor.

One delightful place he went to as a locum for three consecutive summers was Owston Ferry in Lincolnshire. The practice extended on both sides of the river Trent. He went his leisurely rounds on foot, and while ferrying himself across the river in a rowing boat on those shining summer mornings, he decided that the life of a country doctor left little to be desired. It was the country locums which he did at this time which decided him on his future.

Not all his experience was in such pleasant places however. Many months were spent helping out in practices in the industrial towns of the West Riding, including Barnsley, Bradford and Wakefield. These were often practices where half the patients were too poor to pay, and where the doctor had taken on so many patients in order to make a living that his health had broken down, or he had taken to the bottle.

In one practice, the groom had apparently been helping to keep things going as long as possible. He drove Will around and knew all about the patients and what medicines they had. At the end of the first morning he unlocked a small cupboard, brought out a bottle of whiskey and automatically poured out a couple of drinks.

The standards of practice were sometimes deplorably low. Some doctors hardly ever examined their "club" patients, and Will found patients with advanced pulmonary tuberculosis who had been treated with cough mixtures for years, and cases of cancer of the rectum treated with purgatives and never examined.

Before 1911, patients without means and the unemployed and old people whose sole means of support was the old age pension of five shillings a week, called on the "parish doctor" when they were seriously ill. This doctor, whose official title was District Medical Officer, was paid about £50 a year by the Local Authority and usually carried out this work in addition to running his own practice. Not all of them gave the time and care to the destitute and old that they gave to their better-off patients. The next class of patients going up the social ladder was the "club" patient. "Club" patients at that time paid three or four shillings a year, sick or well, to the doctor. Special mixtures compounded of the more economical drugs were provided for them and issued in unwrapped bottles. Above them, in the hierarchy, came the private patients. They had pleasant-tasting and rather expensive flavouring materials added to their medicines, which were issued in wrapped bottles and they were charged "what the traffic would bear". In a city practice, this was usually quite modest, two and sixpence for a visit with perhaps a shilling extra for medicine. It was customary for the doctor to visit his private patients in their homes. When they came to the doctor's house, those above a certain subtle social line were admitted to the doctor's drawing room instead of the surgery, and the doctor's wife would engage them in a few moments' conversation while "the doctor" was being fetched from the surgery.

The District Medical Officer and the Doctors' Clubs did not finally die out until the introduction of the National Health Service in 1948. In 1911 however, soon after Will started in general practice, a major medical reform was introduced by Lloyd George's Liberal government in the form of the National Health Insurance Act. This greatly reduced the proportion of the population dependent on charity or on doctors' clubs for obtaining medical treatment. From then on, the weekly wage earner was "on the panel" and could obtain free general medical treatment. This reform was introduced in spite of much opposition from the medical profession led by the British Medical Association. By a strange trick of history, it was another silver-tongued Welshman, Aneurin Bevan, who thirty-seven years later, in 1948, was to persuade the profession, again much against its will, to complete the work of his predecessor.

The demands of the profession in 1911, as set out by the B.M.A. in six cardinal points, were somewhat unreasonable, including for example that the amount of remuneration must be what the profession considered adequate and that only wage earners with incomes of less than two pounds a week should be entitled to medical benefit. The profession was not solidly behind the B.M.A. as there were many doctors in industrial practices who found it hard to collect fees from the poor people and to make ends meet.

Some leading consultants were conciliatory and Maxwell Telling, a Leeds physician for whom Will had a great regard, wrote a letter to the Yorkshire Post urging that the Council of the B.M.A. should release members from the pledge they had given not to join the scheme. In his letter he said:

"Release from the pledge does not mean approval of the Act; it does not even guarantee support of it; but if such release be given I venture to prophesy that something akin to a shout of joy will go up from the houses of industrial doctors of the Kingdom".

This letter, timed as it was, had a big effect but earned Telling a good deal of unpopularity with the more militant general practitioners who felt that he had betrayed their cause.

Sir John Conybeare,* writing of these events many years later, described the situation as follows:

"At Manchester on December 14th, 1911, the insurgents held a meeting to establish a National Medical Union, the object of which was organised refusal of service under the Bill. The policy of the B.M.A. was denounced as negotiate and procrastinate. Wild scenes of disorder occurred and speakers, including Sir James Barr, who tried to defend the council's action, were howled down. A similar meeting of rebels was held in Birmingham, but the largest and most highly emotional meeting was held at the Queen's Hall in London on December 19th. The hall and galleries were packed long before the meeting started. Stirring music was played on the great organ and as the chairman, Sir Watson Cheyne, came on the platform to the strains of Rule Britannia the audience rose and sang lustily. The platform party included Sir William Osler, Dr. F. J. Smith, and many other consultants. The audience was emotionally labile – roars of applause, shouts of 'No, No', 'Never', cheers and groans. Sir Victor Horsley had a particularly hot reception. Amid shouts of 'traitor', 'Did Lloyd George send you?', he was refused a hearing. Sir William Osler took a poor view of the behaviour of the audience and wrote to the British Medical Journal to that effect . . .

"The appointed day was now only three weeks off. The Christmas truce was barely over when, on January 2nd, 1913, Mr. Lloyd George announced that already nearly 10,000 doctors had joined the panels. In districts where there was a shortage, he said, it might be necessary to close the panels temporarily and install a salaried service. Fortunately these drastic measures never became necessary, as more and more doctors placed themselves on the panel . . .

"The final scene was enacted at the Special Representative

* Sir John Conybeare, "The Crisis of 1911–13, Lloyd George and the Doctors" *Lancet* 1957 1, 1032–5

Meeting on January 18th, 1913, when a motion to release all practitioners from their pledges and undertakings was passed by 115 to 35 divisions. In actual fact a majority of those concerned had already released themselves."

These events were echoed in a remarkable way some thirty-five years later in the controversy which raged around the introduction of the National Health Service. Perhaps the meetings were a little less emotional and the doctors did not sing Rule Britannia, but again there was wide felt anxiety among general practitioners about the possible effects of the extension of Lloyd George's scheme to cover the whole population, not only for general medical services but for all medical services.

Once again, many of the younger (and poorer) doctors were willing to go into the scheme and the consultant leadership by and large supported the government. As in 1911 the B.M.A. resisted the proposed changes, though not so bitterly as they had done on the earlier occasion.

Looking back to 1911, it is easy to attribute the hostility of the medical profession to what was clearly a humane and beneficial reform, to self interest. On the other hand, it should be remembered that apart from the Medical Act of 1858 which ensured an adequate level of training for doctors and established a disciplinary system to prevent or punish "infamous conduct in a professional respect", the profession had been entirely free of state control or interference. Many doctors sincerely believed that the introduction of the government as paymaster for a large section of their patients would impair the trust that should exist between doctor and patient and would bring a free profession under government control.

In the event, the doctors maintained their freedom and a large section of the population, the weekly-wage earners, obtained ready access to general medical advice and treatment without the burden of doctors' bills or the humiliation of charity. In addition, many general practitioners, particularly those who worked in industrial areas and who had for years struggled along on small and uncertain incomes, suddenly found they had financial security. The payment of doctors' bills had always been an uncertain business. The landlord, the grocer, and the publican had to be paid first. If there was a slump, the artisan who fell out of work couldn't pay, and if there was a bad harvest, it was a bad look-out for the country doctor. Then the debt collector would be called in to visit all the patients with unpaid bills, but that too was bad for the practice. A panel of a thousand patients would bring in about four hundred pounds a year, which was at least enough to keep the wolf from the door. Even up to the 1948 Act, Will's income was to some extent affected by the harvest and he would watch the weather at that time of the year with interest and some anxiety.

Will's father, contrary to the views of practically all his colleagues, supported the panel idea. His uncle, Joseph Dobson, on the other hand, refused to go into the scheme until imminent financial ruin forced him to do so. Following the introduction of the scheme, about 800 panel patients enrolled on John Pickles' list, thus assuring him of a fixed basic income.

At about this time Will went as an assistant to Drs. Horsfall and Eddison of Bedale in the North Riding of Yorkshire. This quiet old English town with its massive square church tower looming up at the top of the wide cobbled high street, has changed little over the years.

The practice Will now came to was very up-to-date. It was the first one in which he had worked where the doctor had a telephone and a motor car. Ordinarily Will did his rounds on a bicycle while the partners used the motor, but just occasionally he was able to startle the horses and inhabitants by tearing up the high street at twenty miles an hour in the doctor's new Darracq open two-seater and once, after a severe snowstorm, he went on his rounds for several days in a sledge drawn by a pony and complete with bells.

He lived in a room over a little café; all his expenses were paid and in addition he received five guineas a week, which was a guinea above the usual rate at that time. A few months after he arrived, the senior partner, J. Horsfall, became ill with cancer of the stomach, and Will found himself doing more and more in the practice. He helped in operations carried out on the kitchen table for the removal of the appendix, in the amputation of legs for tuberculosis of the knee joint, and he did most of the midwifery.

It was during the Bedale assistantship that Will's interest in epidemiology was first excited. The incident is best described in his own words:

"A gypsy woman driving a caravan into a village in the summer twilight, a sick husband in the caravan, a faulty pump at which she proceeded to wash her dirty linen, and my first and only serious epidemic of typhoid, left me with a lasting impression of the unique opportunities of the country doctor for the investigation of infectious disease. This incident showed me clearly the ease with which the *fons et origo* of an epidemic could be traced in the country and the simple steps that were sufficient to bring it to an end."

Just as John Snow in 1866 had recommended the authorities to chain up the handle of the Broad Street pump if they wished to end the epidemic of cholera, so Will arranged for this village pump to be put out of commission, and the epidemic of typhoid ended.

Soon afterwards, the young assistant was called to see a case of jaundice which was followed about a month later by quite a crop of similar cases. He had no idea what this infectious disease might be. The senior partner laughed at Will's perplexity and told him not to worry as they all got better. The local "jaundice doctor" who combined this occupation with that of village blacksmith and lamb castrator, recommended the bark of the common berberis, long renowned as a cure for jaundice. Will's self-esteem was slightly restored when he found that some of the most detailed textbooks of the time failed to mention the epidemic nature of this disease. It was then called catarrhal jaundice in the textbooks, but later when its infectious nature was demonstrated, largely by the observations of Will Pickles, it came to be known as infectious hepatitis.

As the months went by, Will became familiar with all the details of the Bedale practice and with the lives of the doctors, the shopkeepers, the farmers and the lowly labourers who cultivated the land with implements which had changed little for centuries. He got to know by heart the bends in the dark lanes of the surrounding countryside and the sombre shapes of the farm buildings as in the night he pedalled wearily home on his bicycle after assisting at the

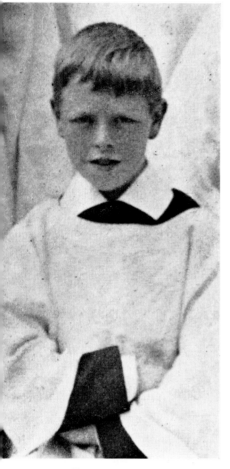 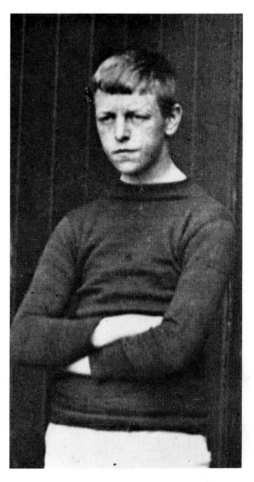

Will as a choirboy   At Leeds Grammar School

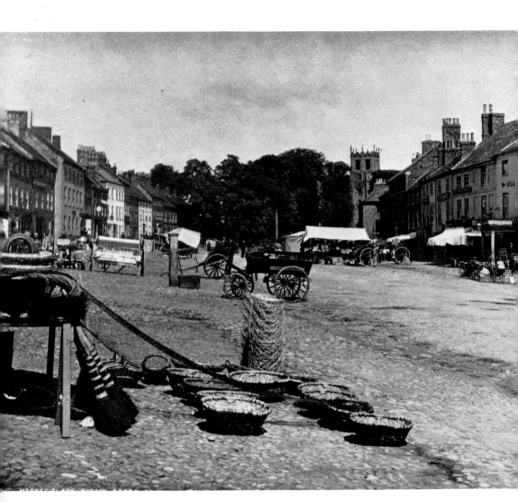

Market place Bedale 1911

entrance of one more human being on to the world's stage, or easing perhaps the exit of another. At these peaceful and solitary times, he would ponder the eternal mystery: "From where do we come? What are we? Whither do we go?" Often he felt lonely and un-settled. He wanted a wife and a home of his own and an established place in society.

There was a settled pattern of social life in Bedale before the First World War. On Sundays, he would be invited to supper at the house of one of the principals or to the rectory. An invitation to the Edisons' house included a bath before dinner and afterwards they would gossip about the practice or play games like Consequences. Sometimes he would receive an invitation to dine with "the County". He did not enjoy these dinner jacket events. Somehow, in spite of their gracious behaviour, you were too often reminded of Lady Chettam's remark in *Middlemarch*: "For my own part, I like a medical man more on a footing with the servants; they are often all the cleverer."

Once a year, Lord B. gave a large garden party with all the grace and condescension possible to a noble family. On one evening a week Will played bridge with two bank managers and a lawyer and sometimes his brother Philip or his parents would come and stay with him.

I visited Dr. Eddison in 1957. He was then nearly eighty, still living in the same large red house in Bedale where Will had gone to Sunday supper forty-seven years before. Although partially paralysed, he was still seeing an occasional patient. He was a big man with a fine countenance, marked with suffering. He described himself as "an old-fashioned liberal with conservative tendencies", and as he sat talking of the years before the First World War, his face was from time to time momentarily contorted with pain and he gripped the sides of his chair. He paid little attention to these spasms but after a pause continued.

"Will's father? Oh yes, he was a dear old boy, and Will, he was an extraordinarily likeable chap, got on well with his patients and a great one for keeping statistics and records and so on. He's been very good on the Local Executive Committee – persuasive and tactful. I don't think he's got any enemies in the district. . . ."

D

Will had hardly been in the Bedale practice a year when Dr. Horsfall died. Will was thereupon invited to buy his way into the practice, but although the terms were favourable, he could not raise the money.

In the days when the buying and selling of practices was the normal way of filling a vacancy caused by the death of a principal, the ability to pay the sum asked by the doctor's widow was usually the most important qualification required of the incoming doctor, providing of course that his name could be found on the Medical Register. In this case, when someone appeared who could raise the money, he was accepted as the new partner, and it was decided to run the practice without an assistant, so Will found himself without a job and once again on the locum market.

In August 1912 he was engaged by Dr. Hime, a man of thirty-five years of age, practising in the village of Aysgarth. Thus Will first came to work in the place where he was to spend the major part of his life. He had in fact, been offered an assistantship in this practice three years before by his cousin, Jo Dobson, the Leeds surgeon, acting on behalf of Dr. Hime. Will had turned it down then as he had wanted to see something of the world before settling down in country practice. He had, however, passed on the offer to his friend of student days, Dean Dunbar, though advising him not to accept it. He told Dunbar that he was too inexperienced and that he would never leave if he did decide to go.

"Damn it, I'll have a flap at it," Dunbar had said, and he stayed there until he died.

"His decision for himself was right," wrote Will. "He loved the place, he loved the people, and never regretted the step he had taken."

When Will arrived at Aysgarth as a temporary assistant, he found that Hime was drinking heavily while Dunbar did most of the work.

Hime was an example of the tragedy which sometimes occurs when a man of high intellectual powers is unable to discover a satisfying outlet for his talents. That he had considerable ability is shown by the fact that he qualified at the early age of twenty-one. He came to Aysgarth at twenty-three and built up the Aysgarth practice from almost nothing. His patients had the sort of faith in him which persuaded them that his skill was of so high an order that even when the worse for drink he was twice as good as any ordinary doctor sober.

Will, although not without experience of this sort of situation, was shocked to see Hime help himself to half a tumblerful of neat whisky from the tantalus before breakfast. He was, however, delighted to be with his old friend Dunbar again and together they began to think how delightful life would be if this practice were theirs. But the locum soon ended and Will went away to do still more locums. He began to despair because without capital he could not get started. He took a locum at Ripon and then went home and did one for his father, so that his parents could get away for a holiday.

Restless and discontented, he determined to get away from Yorkshire for a time at least and to see something of the world. He obtained the post of ship's doctor on the *City of London*, a liner carrying three hundred first-class and one hundred second-class passengers to Calcutta. He joined the ship at Glasgow in October 1912, and had a friendly reception from the ship's officers. Indeed, one of them tried to borrow some money from him even before the ship left dock – a forlorn hope, as he had none. He received a salary of twelve pounds a month from the shipping company which provided a medical service free of charge to the passengers. The passengers made full use of it and a tiresome group was always demanding attention for sea-sickness and other minor or imaginary complaints. There was, however, serious work to be done as well. One member of the crew broke his leg a few days after they had put to sea, and the quartermaster began to cough up blood and had to be put ashore at Tilbury. The *City of London* called at Marseilles, and there Will enjoyed his first experience of foreign travel as he sat and watched the plane trees flickering in the autumn sun, and sipped strange-tasting aperitifs in a little restaurant in the old port. The next call was Port Said. Here a caricaturist whom Will asked to draw him for a joke, said he could find nothing very characteristic to depict about his appearance, except for his red ears.

The ship sailed on to Colombo where Will was fascinated by the great gems displayed in the jewellers' shops, by the steamy atmosphere and the indescribable aroma of the strange and teeming city and by the red road that led to Mount Lavinia.

They reached their destination, Calcutta, in December and Will found it a delightful place to be in; dining at the Bengal Club, dancing at the Saturday Club, attending race meetings, polo matches and the weddings of two or three of the passengers occupied his time, and the horrors of the poverty and disease in that city do not seem to have impressed themselves upon him at all.

During the voyage home, after the passengers' medical needs had been satisfied, the time was occupied with bridge or helping in the entertainments. The handsome young ship's doctor was popular and would help to amuse the passengers at the evening concerts by singing sentimental ballads like The Devout Lover or "naughty" ditties such as The Twins which he sang with a brother officer. And as the ship rolled softly on in the darkness, across the Indian Ocean, the following song might have been heard coming from the passengers' saloon, rising above the tinkle of glasses and the sound of laughter:

1st Twin: "I treat a lady with respect",
2nd Twin: "And I treat her with wine".
1st Twin: "I go down on my knees to her",
2nd Twin: "And I take her on mine".

There was one especial lady on board, a beautiful creature, who quite captured the surgeon's heart, but alas, when the voyage ended, she decided after all to marry a Greek merchant.

In January 1913 he went back to Aysgarth and joined Dunbar again as Hime's second assistant.

4

THE AYSGARTH PRACTICE BEFORE
WILL'S TIME

THE AYSGARTH PRACTICE to which Will now came to spend the rest of his life dates back to about 1860. Before then, the doctor for this part of Wensleydale lived at West Burton. On the green of this beautiful village can still be seen the stocks whose last occupant, it is said, was in fact the local doctor who had been placed there in a state of alcoholic stupor.

Matthew Willis, M.D. Edinburgh, was the first doctor to reside at Aysgarth. He must have been an intelligent man. Will records that he was once shown a mahogany case of surgical intruments awarded to Willis as a prize. The memory of one dramatic event which occurred in the 1860s was described to Will by an old man who had been an eye witness. A workman blasting in the Redmire quarry suffered a severe abdominal injury from an explosion. A man was sent on horseback to find Willis, who was eventually tracked down at the White Hart in Hawes. He told Willis that the poor man's "puddings" (intestines) had been blown out and were "lying agin t'wall". Willis rode about twelve miles to the scene of the accident, pushed the intestines back, stitched up the wound and mounted the man on his own horse and took him home. Miraculously he recovered.

Willis died of tuberculosis in 1871. He was visiting a patient on horseback one day when he suddenly coughed up a large quantity of blood. He just managed to ride home, but never got up from his bed again. He was much loved by his patients, who on his death subscribed to a memorial for him. This took the form of a stained glass window in the parish church. Underneath are inscribed the words:

"Matthew Willis, M.D. died at Aysgarth,
February 1871, aged 43 years. He was a
skilful and distinguished member of his
profession, kind to all, especially to the
poor".

Willis' successor was a Quaker, Richard Laycock Routh, who
seems to have been a likeable character. A letter from him when he
was a medical student in London to his aunt and uncle in Wensleydale recreates a long past Christmas:

"I shall think of you going out in a great troupe at night, tramping
away through the snow almost knee deep and then stopping at
some out-of-the-way farmhouse. There you will strike up a song,
upon which the good people will rush out and bring hot milk,
cheesecakes and all the good things which the Wensleydale people
alone know how to make. These you will have to partake of to
keep the cold out and then the money-box is produced and having
heard the rattle of the money which is dropped in, you say, 'Good
night' and hurry off to perform at some other house and again will
meet with a Wensleydale reception."

In another letter to his aunt and uncle he writes with charming
candour:

"I am no longer best man in anatomy, five or six men have gone
by me. I shall stay here till Christmas and make up my reading
tremendously hard afterwards."

After further reflection he reassures himself:

"Still I think I am far away the best man of my year in many
practical points, especially midwifery and I expect I could diagnose
and treat a case of surgical accident or of disease better than most."

Routh only stayed for about three years in Aysgarth. He married
his housekeeper, the niece of the village blacksmith, and went to
practise elsewhere.

He was succeeded by Alfred Baker who had started practising at
Askrigg but moved to Aysgarth after Routh's departure in about
1874, realising that this was a better centre for practice in the dale.

Baker, like Willis, was loved and respected by the dale folk. He died of dropsy in 1903 at the age of fifty-five, and is commemorated by a brass tablet in the parish church and another in the village institute. He fought for the institute against great opposition and himself contributed fifty guineas towards it, about all he had in the world.

On one occasion he asked Squire Tomlinson for a donation towards it but received a curt refusal to which he replied with spirit: "Damn you, Squire, we'll have an Institute when you're in Hell."

"The Institute" still plays an important part in the life of the village. Downstairs are a billiard room and a committee room, and upstairs a hall where dances are held and occasional meetings such as those of the Wensleydale Society. Once a fortnight the County Library arranges for books to be exchanged there. High up on the wall of the ill-lighted vestibule and almost impossible to read, is the bronze tablet which says:

> "In memory of Alfred Baker, M.R.C.S., L.R.C.P. Born February 18th 1848, died February 7th 1903, who resided at Aysgarth for upwards of thirty years. He was an active supporter of the movement for providing a new Reading Room in the village and a generous subscriber to the building fund. The balance of the money raised by public subscription to provide a suitable memorial to him was paid by the Trustees towards the expenses of erecting this Institute."

Baker was also responsible for getting the present handsome stone "doctor's house" built. He first lived in a more humble house but one day boldly asked the Squire to build him a more fitting house. "You shall have one, and a surgery too," said the Squire, and the present doctor's house with the little surgery annexe was completed in 1889.

The Squire's generosity was somewhat capricious as the following story indicates.

James and Mrs. Winn were walking down to Church one Sunday morning with the Squire. James said, "It's a good object for the collection, Squire, Leeds Infirmary. I'll put a sovereign in if you will." "Aye, it is a good object," said the Squire, "I will." James was Churchwarden and he saw two gold sovereigns in the count and assumed the Squire had kept to his bargain.

As he and his wife returned he said, "The old boy kept his word. There were two sovereigns in the collection." "But," said Mrs. Winn, "I put one in, so there should have been three." Next market day, at Leyburn, James tackled the Squire. "Ay," he said, "you're right, me hand came on a half sovereign and I thought that would do, but it *is* a good object, I wouldn't mind giving £500 to it," and straightway he proceeded to the bank and arranged for this to be done.

"Squire Tomlinson" was the last man in Aysgarth to be given that title, and the old men still talk of him with affection. The local characters would compete to occupy "the Squire's seat" in the George and Dragon before he arrived for his evening drink. When the Squire came in, the occupier of the seat would offer, very courteously, to give it up to the Squire, and was invariably rewarded with a drink.

The Squire often came in with an old village character – Decimus Durham, who lived alone in a cottage farther up the village. He made a habit of teasing Decimus by saying after the first drink: "Well, Des, it's time we were going." "Aye, Squire, so 'tis," said Decimus, but always sat fast until a second round was forthcoming. Decimus sold ha'pennyworths of snuff and he used to walk miles picking up wool from the thorn bushes, spin his own yarn and knit it into socks.

With no television, radio or cinema the country people were obliged to create their own pastimes. Practical jokes provided one of the commonest amusements, and Decimus Durham seems to have been a natural victim. Not only did the occasion itself provide a relief from the monotony of the daily toil, but the repetition of the story afterwards over a garden wall or in the George and Dragon, with suitable embellishments, gave much pleasure. They would tell how some lads had climbed on to the roof of Des's cottage and let a live hen down the chimney on a piece of string, how another had dropped a handful of pepper in Des's ham frying on the range when the old man's back was turned, or another had popped a live pigling through the window at dead of night. Half a century later, long after their subject was dead, these oft-repeated tales still entertained visitors to the dale.

One of the greatest practical jokers, William Winn, lived in Askrigg. He once got an old man drunk at the Kings Arms and then bet him five pounds he couldn't undress in five minutes. The old fellow took the bet on and managed well until he was stuck with taking off his boots. "Cut tha wangs" (bootlaces), said the practical joker, handing him a knife which the victim used, and won his bet. He was then paid by a "cheque" written on a telegraph form, his clothes thrown on to a high shelf in the tap room and the bell loudly rung for the barmaid, who came in, screamed and rushed off for the landlord.

This joker did not always come off best. On one occasion he ordered a glass of whisky and then accused the landlady of watering it.

"You taste it," he said to one of the villagers. The man took a sip and then drank the lot.

"I can see nowt wrang wi' it," he said.

Another source of entertainment was the annual village feast, and Redmire feast was famous. It was held at the end of September on the village green. There were roundabouts with their steam organs blowing, and stalls with brightly coloured striped awnings. People who had moved away from the village returned to see their friends and relations. It was the holiday of the year. There were quoits and skittles competitions, trotting matches and races, and a greasy pole competition with a live pig as a prize for the one who climbed it first. Leyburn Fair was another great occasion. Some would ride in dog carts from the surrounding villages, but many would walk distances of eight or nine miles. From early morning, the roads were full of people and there was company all the way. These feasts would last for four days, there were no licensing hours, and some would not return home until the end. As an old village philosopher said to me: "They got oblivious for a bit and rested their faculties."

The agricultural shows were sometimes held in conjunction with the village feast. On the long trestles in the tents, the exhibits of vegetables and flowers, jams, honeycombs and cakes would be arranged then as today, and excite admiration or envy. Round the ring outside the washed, sleek cattle paraded in front of the judges, and nearby some quack would offer a cure for rheumatism.

The winter was "a long patch of drear" relieved for the older women by quilting parties, when a number of women would meet in someone's house to make a patchwork quilt for a young girl's wedding. For the men, there might be the Rent dinners given once or twice a year by the great landowners to tenants paying more than a certain rent. For the younger generation there were occasional dances at "the Institute" in the winter, but these did not become common until after the First World War.

A vivid picture of country practice in Baker's time is given by Will's published account of the history of the practice[28] in which he describes the recollections that Baker might have had as he lay dying:

"He felt he had lived at a difficult time in medicine. He had been taught good, sound stuff at Mary's. He could set a broken limb with anybody and no one in his hospital days thought much of that Quaker fellow in Glasgow with his fantastic ideas and his claim to have healed compound fractures by first intention with the help of that foul-smelling stuff of his. Now, a German had invented a machine by which you could actually look through the flesh and see the bones. In a way, he felt he had not needed it. He had relied on the touch of his sensitive fingers and a keen eye for alignment; and then he took infinite trouble. One had to live with one's failures as well as one's successes in a country district, and, ah yes, there had been one at least of the former. The postman who limped about his rounds was a living reproach to him, but that was only one failure among so many successes, and he wondered whether those who followed after, even with the help of these Roentgen rays, would have a better record. He thought of the succession of young assistants and how he used to defer to their more recent experience. The patients used to tell them: 'Dr. Baker thinks ye know more than he does, but we don't.' Of course they were all ardent Listerians, and after all Lister was now a Lord so there must have been something in what he said. These lads boiled their instruments and stitches, and scalp wounds and those nasty gashes in arm and leg from the hay field healed in no time and without the intervention of laudable pus which had so often been the fate of his efforts; but they still called him in for his advice and his clever manipulations in midwifery cases, and he knew he could handle those forceps even now and deliver a poor woman when others had failed . . . He thought of bowling along in his smart gig, when it was too hot to ride, or in winter gliding over the snow with all the glamour of sleigh and bells, himself in that warm fur coat old Dives had pressed upon him when he pulled his son through double pneumonia . . . But he had his recreations. He could always spend a few hours down by the stream and go home with a good basket of trout, and those days on the moors after driven grouse, weren't they good? In his heart he still preferred to walk up the birds alone with his dog, and his greatest joy of all was in that marshy land, the 'Strands' by the river where he could almost always fell a 'jack' or a 'full' snipe, and he fancied himself at snipe and woodcock.

"This young fellow Hime who seemed likely to succeed him was tip-top, a regular thruster with good theory and practice. Why, he actually had a surgeon over from Leeds, a likeable youngster with thinning reddish hair and keen clear eyes, some weeks ago. He came on the last train to see a lad with inflammation of the bowels, and with only a paraffin lamp for light and the kitchen table to operate on, these two had removed his vermiform appendix and the lad was now back at work. How he had dreaded those inflammations of the bowel. So many of them recovered in time with linseed poultices and a dose of castor oil, but some slipped through his fingers, and now this young fellow said they should be operated on. Of course, he knew this. When he came into practice first, he was an assiduous reader of his journals. He had tried to keep up-to-date and had read at intervals of this procedure, but the application had not been easy.

"His long after-dinner talks with this assistant over the modest two glasses of '68 had shown him how he had lost touch."

Baker was a wit, and it is recorded that on his death bed he was roused by his housekeeper to ask if he would see the vicar. He declined the visit with the words: "No, I only deal with the Head of the firm." There are still those alive in Wensleydale who remember well the Pickwickian Baker, and recall how he would take a gun with him in the gig on his rounds and how he would be followed by three or four of his beloved dogs ready to retrieve the pheasant or snipe the doctor might bring down between one patient and the next.

After Baker's death in 1903, Edward Hime became the principal. Within a few years, the practice had doubled and Hime bought himself a Darracq motor car. He took some delight in giving the villagers a lift and scaring them by bowling along at twenty miles an hour or so. On one such occasion when he asked a villager if he were frightened, he received the calm reply, "It's thy bloody neck as well as mine, doctor." On another occasion, an elderly gentleman, still living, tells how he was riding home from a meet of the harriers one day, when the red monster came speeding round a bend of the narrow lane. Hime's usual method of stopping in emergencies by changing into reverse gear failed. The car went into the ditch and the horse jumped over the hedge.

Hime had worked with Baker for a few years before the latter's death and had learned a lot from him on how to run a practice. He was energetic and enterprising in his early years as principal and was liked by his patients.

At that time there were no patients in Preston-under-Scar, a village some seven miles to the east of Aysgarth, but one day Hime was called to see a sick woman there. He visited her every day and continued to do so long after it was necessary. After each visit, he would call at the inn for a drink to make himself acquainted with the villagers.

Thus his charm and diligence became known and he acquired many more patients in that village. For a long time after, the first lady patient would blandly say to him: "I was your advertisement, wasn't I, doctor?"

Hime brought to the practice knowledge of the recent advances in surgery. This was the time when it was becoming possible to differentiate between different causes of acute abdominal pain. Appendicitis could now be accurately diagnosed and the offending organ removed by a surgical operation. Thus Hime introduced the idea of sending for a surgeon for these acute abdominal emergencies and the operations would usually be performed on the kitchen table. If this were at night, a collection of candles and hurricane lamps would be assembled to illuminate the operation. If a surgeon could not be obtained from Leeds, Hime himself would operate. On these occasions, the chloroform would be administered by his assistant. George Cockcroft, a neighbouring doctor, recalled how he was once called to see a patient by an old doctor at Hawes. He found a strangulated hernia and said, "Will you give the anaesthetic, or do the operation?" The Hawes doctor scratched his head and said he'd never seen an anaesthetic given. The patient, hearing the conversation, burst in, "Let's not bother wi' chloroform. Get on with the operation and put me out of this pain," and so they did and the patient made a good recovery.

Hime found in his midwifery practice that he was up against some powerful traditions. He insisted on cleanliness, though the custom then was for the woman in labour to retain her used night clothes and even her day clothes for the confinement. The handywoman who had been engaged by the young mother or grandmother would often say to Hime: "Can't you give her something, doctor, to help her?" meaning ergot which Baker invariably gave but which Hime had been taught was dangerous. He often did not see the patient until called to the confinement by the handywoman. Sometimes the date of delivery was hopelessly wrong and the handywoman would say: "Ay, she's laid her cinders wrong" – referring to the custom followed by illiterate mothers of laying a cinder on the mantelpiece for each missed period.

In spite of their lack of cleanliness and the fact that they often sent for him much too early or too late, Hime respected these handy-women who gave up their time and sleep often for no payment to help their fellow village women. They were also the source of endless information about the people among whom he practised, and the gossip would help to relieve the tedium while they waited with a woman in labour.

Hime had had several assistants before Dunbar came in 1910. One, an Irishman like Hime, would occasionally go in the Darracq to

meet Hime at Leyburn station after he had been on a trip to London
or Leeds. On one such occasion, the two doctors called in at several
inns on the way back and finally started to quarrel as to who was in
the best state to drive the Darracq home. They eventually arrived
back at Aysgarth in the small hours, still disputing the question. They
thereupon took off their coats and started fighting in the yard in
front of the surgery. Fortunately they were both keen billiards
players and the following evening were to be found playing billiards
in the Institute as usual.

It is surprising that the round in Hime's day extended even farther
than it does today and included the village of Preston-under-Scar
which lies beyond Redmire. Occasional visits to Hawes in the
opposite direction were also made.

Around 1904 Hime bought out the doctor at West Burton and

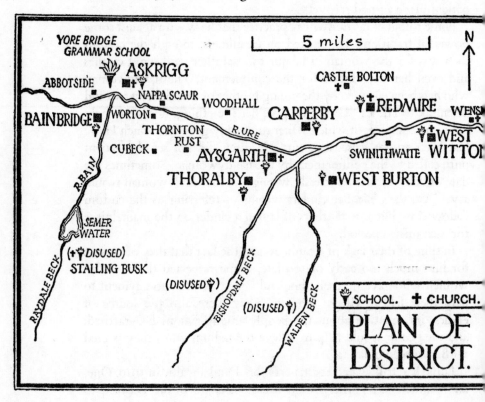

thus created what amounted to a closed area for the Aysgarth practice from Bainbridge up dale to Preston-under-Scar down dale.

Reference to the map opposite shows the extent and main geographical features of the practice. It extends east and west along Wensleydale from West Witton in the east to Bainbridge in the west, a distance of some ten miles as the crow flies. Down the middle of the dale flows the river Ure. From the south, two important tributaries run into the Ure, the Bishopdale Beck, which itself receives the Walden Beck, and to the west the River Bain on the course of which lies the placid lake of Semer Water. From the north, three smaller tributaries enter the Ure as it flows from Bainbridge to West Witton, the Sargill, Cogill and Apedale Becks. Along these little streams and the rivulets that feed them lie the remote farm-houses of the practice. As you climb the fells which rise to nearly two thousand feet on either side of the broad dale the farms become smaller and poorer and the distances between them longer. In the early days, as Will climbed to these lonely farms, perhaps on a cold and rainy night to help some woman in labour, he often thought of the lines of Christina Rosetti:

"And does the road wind up hill all the way?
Yes, to the very end."

On either side of the Ure run the two main routes of the practice. Travelling from the eastern extremity westwards along the top road, the way lies through Redmire, Carperby and Askrigg. After going through Askrigg the road turns south to Bainbridge which marks the western end of the practice. Coming back on the south road it passes through Worton, Aysgarth and West Witton. On the right of this road and to the south can be seen the great flat-topped eminences of Addlebrough and Penhill separated by Waldendale and Bishopdale.

In the length of the practice, there are only four bridges across the river which separates these two roads, and east of the Aysgarth Falls there are none for five miles. This geographical feature has always meant that the round of visits has to be carefully planned beforehand, otherwise a great deal of time is wasted. From the top road and the low road secondary roads run south and north and on these lie the smaller villages of West Burton, Thoralby and Thorton Rust to the south, and Castle Bolton to the north. These secondary roads themselves continue their upward climb to hamlets such as Newbiggin and Countersett before they degenerate into cart tracks to end in the yard of an upland farm.

To the east of the village a road runs down to the Aysgarth Falls by the Palmer Flatt hotel. The road crosses the upper falls where the river changes from its previous quiet flow to a thundering cascade, stained brown with the upland peat when there has been rain, as it drops two hundred feet over the upper, middle and lower falls. These falls in their beautiful wooded setting have made this part of the dale a special attraction for visitors. Sometimes in the summer droughts the water all but dries up and the children paddle in the pools and leap across the river on the hot, dry rocks. In a severe winter the falls freeze into vertical columns of ice against a background of black trees in the deep snow. To the past practitioners of Aysgarth, viewing these scenes from horseback or on foot, perhaps with the snow driving into their faces as they made their way to a patient, the view was not always so much appreciated as it is by the summer visitor. But they were men of determination and good heart and earned the trust and affection of the dales folk who called on them for help.

In Baker's time, the round entailed ten or twelve miles on horseback or in the gig and was in fact usually completed in the morning. If there were an extra number of patients to be seen, the doctor would occasionally have lunch at the local inn, perhaps at Redmire or Askrigg, and finish the visits in the afternoon.

By the time Will arrived in the practice Hime did most of the visiting in the Darracq, but he still kept two or three horses and a trap.

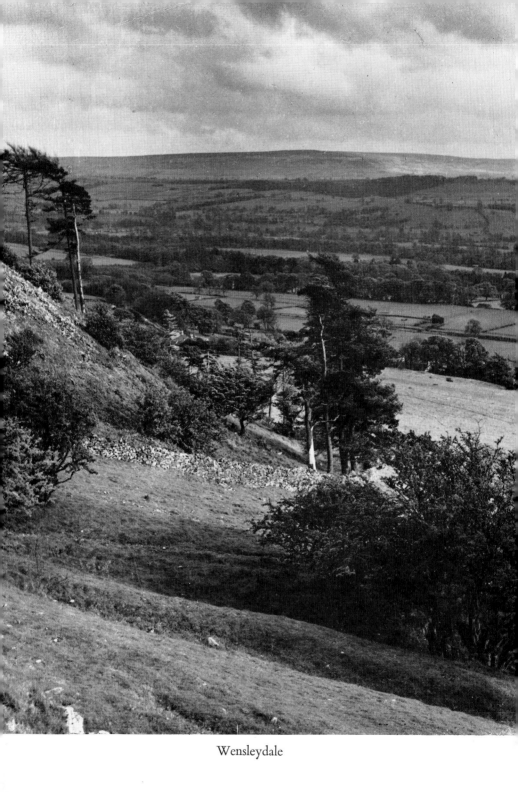

Wensleydale

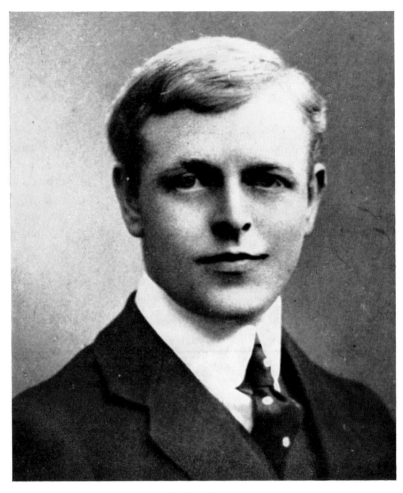

Medical student 1909

5

SETTLING DOWN AT AYSGARTH

DUNBAR WAS DELIGHTED when Will returned to Aysgarth after his voyage to India, and the two friends did a round together the next day on horseback. Will was happy to be back – he knew and liked Dunbar and he knew Hime. He settled into the work immediately. His salary was four guineas a week and all found. He lived with the other two doctors in the big stone house that Squire Tomlinson had built for Baker. All three were bachelors. Hime was a man of charm and a noted lady-killer and he could manage the patients. He came from an old Irish family and "didn't give a damn" for the wealthy ones. "They're not in the stud book and I am," he would say. He was much respected as a doctor and the older inhabitants of the dale still talk of him with relish and affection. Although he occasionally called in a consultant from Leeds, he tackled nearly everything himself, difficult midwifery cases and emergencies of all kind. As the old retired "postie" put it to me: "He would have considered it lowering to his dignity not to have been able to deal with the sort of cases you chaps send off to hospital today."

Very soon after Will had arrived, he and Dunbar began to consider how they might bring Hime to the point of selling the practice to them as he had promised. Hime was then only thirty-five, but had lost interest in general practice and was also finding the attentions of a young woman, who had certain claims upon him, to be an embarrassment. He was therefore not unwilling to leave the district. So one evening after dinner, the three of them with their lawyer and accountant drew up and signed a provisional agreement by which Hime was to receive a thousand pounds down, and two hundred a year for ten years. Will knew he would find it hard to raise his share of the purchase price of the practice, but eventually a wealthy friend of the lawyer called in to complete the transfer invested five hundred pounds in the practice, his cousin Dr. Jo Dobson lent him two hundred, and a consultant at Leeds fifty pounds. Dunbar raised the rest.

Hime decided to sever his ties in Wensleydale once and for all, and to emigrate to Canada. "Tell her I'm drinking and not fit to marry anyone," he said to Will. In March 1913, barely two months after Will had arrived in Aysgarth, he accompanied Hime to Leeds and tried to get him into an hotel. Hime, however, was so drunk that the hotel refused to take him. Finally, after much trouble, Will got him into an obscure hotel, and the next day arranged for him to be admitted to a nursing home. Hime never got to Canada and later, when Will had occasion to visit him, he found him, his hands stained with French polish, working as a clerk and odd job man in a cheap furniture firm in Leeds. When the 1914 war came, Hime rang up the War Office about an invention he had worked out to bomb the Germans from the air. Later he had a mental breakdown and was admitted to a mental hospital. He recovered in a short while, joined up, served in Serbia and was appointed medical adviser to the Serbian Ministry of Health for which he received a decoration. After the war, his life assumed a steadier course. He married and settled down in general practice again in Yorkshire. He had overcome his alcoholism by this time. He died in 1934 at the age of fifty-nine.

Will's partnership with Dean Dunbar was a happy one. It endured from 1913 until Dunbar's death at the age of fifty in 1935. Dunbar was an ideal partner. There was complete trust between the two doctors and they never had a serious quarrel. "A successful partnership," wrote Will, "so like a successful marriage, is founded on mutual trust as well as mutual affection and that is what made those twenty-two years so pleasant and profitable to ourselves and by those tokens to our patients." He did not mean profitable in a financial sense, for elsewhere he notes: "I do not regret it and although the income has never been large I would not have spent my life elsewhere for twice the sum. I took to the people and I believe they took to me."

Dunbar was a taciturn man and it is said that he would sometimes enter a patient's bedroom with a curt nod, make a careful examination without a word and leave with another nod and never a word. And yet eventually his genuine kindness and conscientiousness made him one of the most popular figures in the dale. There was never any jealousy between him and Will, and if either was puzzled by a case they would go back and see the patient together. When Dunbar did speak he spoke with force. A young neighbouring doctor once said to the two partners, "I love pneumonias." After he had gone Dunbar turned to Will and said, "If he'd seen as many die as we have he'd think as we do and it's a damned, dirty, bloody, disease; and he will."

This was many years before the discovery of sulphonomides and antibiotics. The only treatment for pneumonia then was tepid sponging and good nursing. Village people would sometimes kill a young rabbit, skin it and apply the skin while still warm to the affected side of the sufferer's chest.

On one occasion Dunbar was driving a serious-minded relative in his motor bike and sidecar rather fast round the winding lanes near West Burton when he had to swerve violently to avoid a horse and cart. On recounting it the relative said it was only the hand of God that saved them. "Ay," interposed Dunbar, "and a bit of bloody good steering." He would spend hours crouching down by his motor cycle trying to improve its performance, quietly talking and chuckling with the local garage hand.

Dunbar had a remarkable memory for all the details of his patients' lives and illnesses but he never made a note. Perhaps this was as well as his writing was illegible. Later on Will persuaded him to dictate his notes while Will recorded them in longhand. These were of considerable value for subsequent reference as he had a keen clinical eye and "intensely choice language." He also had great practical ingenuity. Once when he had been summoned to a remote farm to see an unfortunate woman who was dying of cancer of the breast, he found she had retention of urine due to spinal metastases. He would have had a long walk back to the village to get the catheter that was needed, but while looking out of the window he saw some geese in the yard. He asked the farmer to fetch a goose's quill.

He fashioned it into a serviceable catheter which was then boiled and used to give the patient relief.

After Hime's departure, Will and Dunbar continued to live in "the doctor's house", and the first year at Aysgarth was one of the happiest of Will's life. They had two maids to wait on them and Matt Sayer, who had previously worked for Hime, was manservant and groom. They had coal fires in their bedrooms in the winter and lived well in spite of the rigours of the climate. They told the cook they did not like "made up dishes" and enjoyed a hot roast on six days a week. They enjoyed entertaining their friends and relatives lavishly.

There was a much greater difference between the standard of living of the prosperous middle classes and manual workers at that time than there is today. Farm labourers were paid eighteen shillings a week and some had "butcher's meat" only twice a year, at Christmas and at the Aysgarth feast. The staple diet was bread, potatoes and bacon.

By listening to the tales of the old patients still living when he went there in 1911, Will was able to form a picture of life in the dale in the middle of the nineteenth century. Without any social security other than the workhouse or outdoor relief, it was often a sad picture that was recalled. An old lady, Alice Chapman, told him that as a maid she got one shilling a week as wages. When she was fourteen she was able to buy her first pair of leather shoes, having worn only wooden clogs till then. She had brought up a family of step-children in the 1850s. Often there was no food in the house and when the children were crying with hunger she used to put the "back-stean girdle" on the fire and by pretending there was food to come, pacify them and send them to sleep.

Some of the older inhabitants of Aysgarth can remember Will's arrival. Unlike Dunbar, who looked older than his years, Will looked remarkably young. The older farmers at first would say: "Ah'm not takking ony notice o' him, he's nobbut a bit o'a lad." However, what he and Dunbar lacked in experience, they made up for in conscientiousness and energy. Will enjoyed the great satisfaction of feeling that the patients were his, and his confidence increased as he found that he could usually deal effectively with the various illnesses which were presented to him. When the problem was too difficult he could call in the sturdy and taciturn Dunbar to advise, or at least to share the burden of anxious uncertainty, and for patients who were plainly very ill and in whom the diagnosis was in doubt or for whom surgical treatment was required, one of their old teachers from Leeds could be summoned.

In the case of a surgical emergency they sent for Will's cousin Joe Dobson, a surgeon on the staff at Leeds General Infirmary. He always came cheerfully if he possibly could, although the fee was never large and sometimes uncertain. Will would try and arrange some recreation for him such as a shoot on the Strands, and he usually took a pheasant or two back with him to Leeds.

Tuberculosis was a great killer in those days and there was no effective treatment. Isolation of the infectious case in a sanatorium was the main method of preventing its spread, but this was by no means always successful as Will once recorded:

"Almost forty years ago, when I entered my present practice, one Sunday afternoon my partner and I set off on horseback to visit certain remote farms which he was anxious to show me and which were only attainable by that method of transport. In one of the most remote of these a man sat crouched over the fire. As we talked to him, his thin shoulders were shaken by a dreadful cough and he spat frequently and some of his sputum did not reach the fire. The kitchen seemed to be filled with dark, curly-headed little girls and we chased them away whilst we stripped our patient for examination. The signs were unmistakable. We carried back his sputum in an old Bovril jar and late though was the hour of our return, stained and examined it, the diagnosis was only too easy. That man is living at the age of seventy-nine today but three of those delightful children died in early womanhood from pulmonary tuberculosis and a fourth, with a growing family of her own, has signs in her chest and intermittently a positive sputum. The blame rests not with this old man; it rests with ourselves. The public are insufficiently informed on the infectious nature of this most serious of all our infections."

Practically all confinements took place at home and could cause

great anxiety. Describing midwifery in his early days in Aysgarth
Will wrote:

"The present generation of doctors does not realise the toil
maternity was in those days. There were no district nurses and the
doctor was sent for at the first sign. If the house was a 'bye-side
spot', although the birth was in no way imminent, it was less
trouble to stay the night – in bed if this were possible, or in a not
too comfortable chair before the fire. As a rule one was made
much of and one's bodily needs attended to, but I could rarely eat
until the arrival of the babe. Afterwards the superb breakfast,
piping hot from the fire, generally bacon and eggs, was some
compensation for one's vigil.

"There was no ante-natal care and the first intimation was often
the night bell; but with roomy pelves in a ricketless area, it was
surprising how little real trouble there was and how well the
majority fared. In the end Dean and I always called in the other,
when forceps had to be applied."

The fracas which had accompanied the introduction of the
National Health Insurance scheme had died down, and Dean Dunbar
and Will found themselves with a panel of six hundred patients,
which eventually increased to about eight hundred. These provided
a basic income, in addition to what they earned in fees.

The daily routine followed a fixed pattern. The two doctors met
in the tiny surgery at 8·30 a.m. and, each with his visiting book at
hand, reported on the previous day's visits. Mrs. Alderson was
worse and would need visiting again today; she would need some
laudanum. Miss Smith was as usual, pathetically apprehensive and
overflowing with tedious symptoms. She required "a bottle" but
needn't be visited for a week. Mr. Metcalfe had a rash on his
abdomen; could this be typhoid? Each doctor went up dale or down
dale on alternate days, thus every patient had the advantage of seeing
both doctors. Of course, not every patient held the view that two
heads are better than one, and some would come to depend more on
one than the other of the two young doctors. It was rare for a patient
to insist on seeing only one of the partners however, but when this
occurred they did their best to accommodate him or her.

Surgery hours were kept to a minimum and patients were quite content to wait patiently for the doctor's return if he were out on a visit. They were made comfortable in front of a roaring kitchen fire and comforted with cups of tea and cheesecakes provided by the kind-hearted cook.

Medicines were left at the village Post Office or at certain shops to be collected, or occasionally they were sent via a patient from the same village who had come to the surgery. However, they did not always reach their destination, as the following story shows:

John Swinithwaite, a tradesman, came to Aysgarth at Christmas time to collect his accounts. He had one for the doctor, who paid him and gave him some whisky. "Now, John," said the doctor, "will you take these medicines to Witton?" "Aye, sure I will," said John who then had another drink at the George and Dragon. The medicines never reached their destination. The doctor tackled John on this a few days later. "Eh," he said, "I was gwine to tell ye. I was climbing up Temple Bank and I felt rather droughty, so I sat down on a stean and supped the lot and felt better after, and the bottles are over t'wall if ye want them."

Various methods of transport were employed by Will and Dunbar to get up and down the dale to visit their patients. They still maintained two horses and a trap but in addition there was a variety of push-bikes and a single-gear Triumph motor cycle which stood high above the ground. Going up a steep hill it was often necessary to hop off the Triumph and to run along with the engine still going. Not infrequently, Will's coat would get caught in the driving belt bringing man and machine ignominiously to the ground. The remainder of the visits had then to be completed with bruised knees and bleeding hands. Sometimes he went round on a push-bike, but this was a slow and arduous means of transport in this hilly district. On afternoon visits he generally travelled on horseback and he would stable the horse at the Rose and Crown in Bainbridge while visiting patients in the village.

There was one mare called Topsy which crawled like a slug on the outward journey, but would fly on the road home. As soon as she realised the last visit had been completed, she would break into a gallop before Will was properly in the saddle, and on one occasion

threw him in the ditch as she made off homewards. Fortunately a
road man intercepted her and, encouraged with a shilling, promised
to keep the whole incident a secret.

On one occasion Dunbar was riding a spirited mare called Dolly,
and wished to take a short-cut home across the river by the stepping
stones. Hime had previously told him never to let Dolly stop and
drink from the river. However, the horse seemed so tired and docile
when they came to the river that Dunbar allowed her to stop for a
drink. When he thought she had had sufficient, he tried to get her
head away from the water by pulling sharply on the bridle. Dolly
resented this and showed it by rearing back on her hind-legs,
casting the good natured Dunbar backwards into the river. She then
galloped home, leaving the dripping doctor to follow. Hime, a true
Irishman, had loved his horses, and was a master in the saddle even
when the worse for drink. Neither Will nor Dunbar had the
gift. As Matt Sayer put it, long after: "They warn't very good
jockeys."

When the horses finally went, after the First World War, that
picturesque figure the doctor's man was also dispensed with. They
used to be known by the name of the doctor, "Will Baker's" or
"Matt Hime's". In the early years, Will occasionally combined the
railway with the bicycle to carry out his rounds as economically as
possible. He would cycle up or down the dale with the prevailing
wind, and carry out visits on the way. He would then put the bicycle
in the guard's van and take the train back to the other extremity of
the practice, for example from Wensley to Askrigg, and then cycle
back to Aysgarth, again with the wind behind him and visiting
patients *en route*. Many visits were made at night to the remote farms
and cottages for some emergency, and at such times the local ghost
stories, of which there were many, would often come to mind.

Sometimes their horses would start and quicken their pace at these
places as if they were affected by some "perturbèd spirit".

A place near Ribblehead was said to be haunted by the ghost of a
little girl affectionately known as Little Peg. She would be found
crying and wringing her hands, and would jump up and seat herself
by the carter on his way home in the dusk. Everyone loved her and
was not in the least afraid. She seemed always to be looking for

something. At about this time a gun in one of the butts at Gearstones saw something shining in the mud. This turned out to be a Roman bangle and it was suggested that this being found (it is now in the British Museum) her spirit is at rest.

There was no public road conveyance in or out of Aysgarth before the First World War. A wagonette could be hired at the George and Dragon and this was used for meeting people at the station or for an outing to Leyburn. The village people travelled about very little beyond the range of their legs or a pony cart. The railway was used mainly by summer visitors and the gentry, and only rarely by the poorer people, when a longer journey was imperative. This limitation on travelling in the dale had an important bearing on the researches which Will later undertook as it helped him to trace the source and spread of a new epidemic.

During the next forty years, a network of bus services developed which today allows cheap and easy communication between the villages. Day trips bring coach loads of visitors from Leeds and other industrial towns into the dale on summer Sundays, and many other tourists come in cars to see the Falls. The railway was increasingly neglected after the Second World War. The passenger trains travelled with fewer and fewer coaches until finally the train consisted of only one coach carrying a handful of passengers at hopelessly uneconomic rates. Around 1953 this little line from Northallerton to Hawes was finally closed to passenger traffic.

When Will started in Wensleydale only the main roads were macadamised. The secondary roads to the outlying villages were rough and dusty in the summer and quagmires in the winter, while the hamlets and farms could be reached only along rough tracks on foot or on horseback. Even today, it may be impossible in winter to take a car within a quarter of a mile of some of the upland farms.

Because of the scattered nature of the Aysgarth practice, and the difficulties involved for the patients in visiting the doctor, it has always been run largely on the basis of visiting by the doctor rather than attendance at the surgery by the patient. It was not easy for the farmer or farm labourer to call the doctor in an emergency as it would often mean a long trek on foot or horseback to Aysgarth.

Later on, when public telephones were installed in the villages, it was easier to communicate with the surgery at Aysgarth. For a long time Will and Dunbar refused to install the telephone, believing that it might encourage unnecessary calls, and it was not until 1931 that they finally capitulated, largely because the village postmistress was being asked to take so many messages to the doctor. The dalesmen are independent and stoical however, and they appreciate the trouble involved for the doctor in making an extra visit after he has completed his rounds in this sort of country. For these reasons, the Aysgarth doctors know that when they receive a summons for help, it is usually for some serious illness or accident, or because the birth of a baby is imminent.

In October 1913, Dunbar married Kathleen Downham, a parson's daughter from Liverpool. Will very much wanted to go to Liverpool for the wedding, but the practice could not be left, and so he had to fulfil his role of best man by proxy.

Will stayed on in the doctor's house, living with the Dunbars for a few months, but he soon realised that Dunbar now had a life of his own apart from the practice and his friendship with Will. He therefore moved across to the Post Office about twenty yards distant. Here he occupied two bedrooms and a sitting room. He was awakened with an early cup of tea and his letters at 6.50 a.m. Hot water was carried up in the kettle from the kitchen hob and cold water in a ewer from the stand pipe in the yard. They were then mixed in the round saucer-like bath in which Will splashed about in the middle of the second bedroom. There was no main drainage and the future Medical Officer of Health for this district of the North Riding may have doubted the adequacy of the local sanitation as he contemplated the simple two-seater privy midden that served the inhabitants of the Post Office.

In spite of these minor inconveniences it was delightful to be settled. The practice grew. Soon Dunbar and Will were making a net income of £500 a year each, and with income tax at only a shilling in the pound, they found themselves comfortably established.

Social life flowed freely and pleasantly. They had many friends in whose homes they were welcome. Dinner parties, tennis parties and bridge parties were the chief means by which these social contacts were effected.

Will was often invited to take a glass of sherry or madeira on his round in the morning, but he refused these offers as the round was a long one and took all his time to complete. The owner of one of the big houses, James Winn, showed a friendly attitude from the first. "Treat my home as if it were your father's house," he once said to Will.

"Really country practices were pleasant places in those days," wrote Will much later. "We had lots of friends and a bachelor was made welcome at all the pleasant parties. Nearly everyone had a tennis court and we received more invitations than we were able to accept. The single man was often asked to stay on to dinner and all this made for close friendship."

Subscription dances provided the highlights. These were run by the Badminton club on which centred the social life of the younger generation of ladies and gentlemen. The committee would hire a small orchestra consisting of a piano and a violin and the dance would be held in one of the village institutes. By the rules, alcoholic drinks could not be served in the institutes, but the committee would overcome this difficulty by arranging for a private bar to be set up in a house or shop across the road, where they would drink sparkling burgundy. Sometimes these parties would be held in the big houses, in The Grange at West Burton or at Elm House, Redmire. Will particularly enjoyed visiting Thornton Lodge west of the hamlet of Thornton Rust. This great house had been built in 1909 by a wealthy Burnley mill owner, Mr. Harry Tunstill as a holiday retreat for his family. He had one son and six daughters. The youngest but one was Gerty, and she and Will first met in 1913.

Gerty had spent much time at Thornton Lodge as a child following a severe attack of whooping-cough which left her partially deaf. She had a governess but was allowed to "run wild" on the farm helping with the horses, riding bare back and going to many tennis parties and picnics in the summer.

Her grandfather, who had built up the family business in Burnley, had been a hard working Quaker who went to work at 5 a.m. As a child in Burnley she was often awakened by the clatter of clogs on the pavement. Sometimes she would look out of the window at the stooping men, and the women with dark shawls drawn tightly over their heads, hurrying along to work.

At Thornton Lodge the Tunstills had four housemaids, two pantry maids and a cook, and the children had their own maid. There was also the outside staff of four gardeners and a coachman and grooms. When they went to Scotland for a holiday they rented a shoot near Stonehaven. They hired a special train to carry the twenty-five members of the family and their servants and four horses, and the six girls were allowed to watch the shooting from a waggonette.

Will and Gerty saw a good deal of each other at tennis parties and dances and went riding together. As the New Year, 1914, was rung in, it seemed to Will that all was for the best in the best of all possible worlds. He was twenty-eight, he had achieved his ambition of obtaining a country practice, he was financially secure and he had met someone with whom he hoped to spend his life.

On Sunday, August 2nd, he received a telegram on which was one mysterious word, "Advorcam". He knew that this meant he had to report to H.M.S. *Albion* at Plymouth.

6

THE FIRST WORLD WAR

IN APRIL 1914, Will, with his brother Philip, had joined the Royal Naval Volunteer Reserves.

They had been deeply impressed by a lecture given by Lord Roberts who was travelling up and down the country appealing to young men to join the Reserves. Will was given the rank of Surgeon-R.N.V.R. and an allowance for a uniform. In July, he had taken part in a test mobilisation, but even then the idea that war would shortly come and disrupt his newly-found happiness and security in Wensleydale did not enter his head.

On that first Sunday morning in August, he went round to all the villages with his brother Jack, who had come over to help Dunbar in his absence, saying goodbye to his patients. Many of the villagers to whom Will spoke that morning as they came out of church into the sunshine, or stood in little clumps on the village green, could hardly believe that their friendly young doctor was really going to leave them. To them, this was perhaps the first intimation that something was seriously wrong. To Will the bottom seemed to have fallen out of his world. The afternoon was spent in packing and that night he caught the milk train to Northallerton, and arrived in Plymouth on the morning of Monday, August 3rd.

The *Albion* was an old ship of 12,000 tons, a predecessor of the *Dreadnought*. Its heaviest guns were four twelve-inchers and the ship's crew numbered about 800, of whom most were regulars. He received a heartening welcome from his old shipmates of the R.N.V.R. Later he heard the Articles of War read out, including all the penalties that might be imposed for breaches of discipline, with the ominous phrase: "The penalty for this is death or such penalty as shall be hereinafter mentioned". A cockney seaman standing nearby was heard to remark "Blimey I don't see how I'm going to save my life not no-how."

There were three other surgeons on board, all senior to Will. He found the absence of any but the most trivial medical work difficult to support and was relieved when, after spending ten days in dock taking on stores and equipment, the *Albion* sailed into the English channel to help guard the Expeditionary Force as it sailed across to France. They then sailed to the Bay of Biscay for battle practice. Will felt a strange sense of unreality when after a few days they arrived at Gibraltar as though on a summer cruise. He had been elected wine caterer for the officers' mess and spent pleasant hours wandering around the town in the sun buying quantities of French and Spanish wines. From Gibraltar, the *Albion* proceeded south to the Cape Verde Islands. Here she performed the quiet task of guard-ship for weeks on end. They were allowed ashore, where Will was horrified to find that the local lunatic asylum was open to the public who could go in and watch the lunatics in cages.

It was during this period that he slipped on deck, dislocating a tendon in his leg. In spite of the combined efforts of the three other surgeons on board, the leg remained painful and useless. He was therefore sent back to Gibraltar on a merchant cruiser and the leg put in plaster at the naval hospital. He stayed there for three further months helping in the hospital. Soon after the plaster was removed, the tendon slipped out of place again and finally he was sent home on a P. & O. liner to see Robert Jones, the orthopaedic surgeon, subsequently knighted for his work for the rehabilitation of disabled soldiers. Robert Jones operated on Will, and the tendon was at last securely anchored. He spent his convalescence partly at Leeds with his parents and partly at Aysgarth. During this period he saw much of Gerty.

After two months he was fit, but instead of going back to the *Albion* he was ordered to report to a P. & O. merchant cruiser, the *Macedonia*. They sailed to Cape Verde again, and then were ordered out to sea to patrol the South Atlantic seeking German raiders.

Letters did not travel so swiftly then as they do today, and there was more time for the development of one's feelings between the writing of a letter and its answer. Will had plenty of time to write at length to Gerty as the *Macedonia* lingered at Cape Verde or steamed slowly along the equator. In one of his letters he asked her to marry him, and after the fewest possible number of weeks, he received a favourable reply. This was naturally followed up by a formal letter to her father asking for permission to marry his daughter at some mutually convenient date. Ultimately, this letter too was answered satisfactorily if not enthusiastically, and with an economy of words appropriate to a successful business man:

"Dear Dr. Pickles,
 I can only say I shall put nothing in the way of your happiness.
Yours faithfully,
Harry Tunstill".

Will now wanted desperately to get home, but the *Macedonia* moved out into the South Atlantic again, steaming along at twelve knots in her search for armed merchant-men.

One event that varied the monotony was refuelling under steam from a collier at sea. It was necessary to keep moving to avoid a torpedo from a stray submarine that might have been tracking them. The *Macedonia*'s course took her farther and farther from home; to Rio, Pernambuco, Bahia, Montevideo and Santos. A mildly exciting incident occurred when one of the ship's officers, an inveterate naturalist, brought a female tarantula complete with eggs, on board. The bite of this spider was believed to cause dancing mania and the naturalist was ordered to get rid of it. Will chloroformed the spider, which they then stuffed. On another occasion Will was nearly drowned when the picket in which he was returning from shore leave was swamped by a heavy sea.

Then they had a spell patrolling the River Plate to prevent interned German ships from escaping. Here he spent a day trying to help a Uruguayan lighthouse keeper with gall-stone colic and for his efforts received a document of thanks in flowery terms from the Uruguayan government. In Maldonado at the mouth of the River Plate the British Vice-Consul helped him to find a type of toad described by Darwin in his *Voyage of the Beagle*. They were attractive little creatures with coal-black backs and orange and yellow bellies. Will kept them in a glass covered box on board for many months,

hoping that they would sail home and that he would be able to hand
them over to the London Zoo. This did not happen, however, and
Will, thinking the toads had "not had a square deal", took them
back on a return visit and deposited them in the wood from which
they had come. He also kept an owl in his cabin and fed it on raw
liver. But it too was eventually liberated. Although Will never became a serious naturalist, from an early age he got much enjoyment
from observing birds and mammals.

Apart from lecturing the crew on the dangers of venereal disease
and pulling out a few teeth, there was little medical work to be done.

At Trinidad Island, Will landed with a party, but all they found
was a barren waste populated by land crabs which had destroyed all
the vegetation except the giant tree ferns. Just off the coast lay a
wreck, the *Santa Catarina*, which contained a cargo of sewing
machines. They rowed over the wreck and could uncannily see her
deck quite plainly through the clear water. The ship's divers
recovered some of the sewing machines and made them serviceable.

One of Will's brother officers who had served on the Royal Yacht
endeared himself to Will by his harmless vanity. He would proudly
show him photos taken on his voyages, pointing out members of
the Royal Family. "There is the King, there is the Queen and there's
me," he would say, and after a few drinks he would add, "I know
I'm a snob, I know it, no one better, but there are worse folks than
snobs."

To while away the time, sailing regattas using the ship's boats,
and boxing tournaments were organised, and for a golden sovereign
they could buy a boat load of fresh food from the shore.

The hours of monotony on these slow sea voyages were not
entirely wasted. Will decided to read for his London M.D. He had
a 1901 edition of Osler's *Medicine*, probably the last and best complete text book of medicine in English by a single author. The style
was lucid and the experience of the writer immense. The clinical
descriptions of disease have not been bettered.

At last, at the end of two years, he and his opposite number, a
naval surgeon named Russell, heard they were to be relieved.
Russell with great unselfishness insisted that Will should go first, as
he knew he wanted to get married. This kindly act probably cost

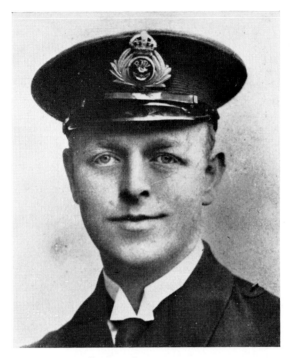

In the Royal Navy 1914–18

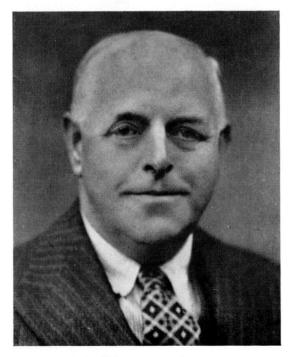

Will in 1935, aged 50

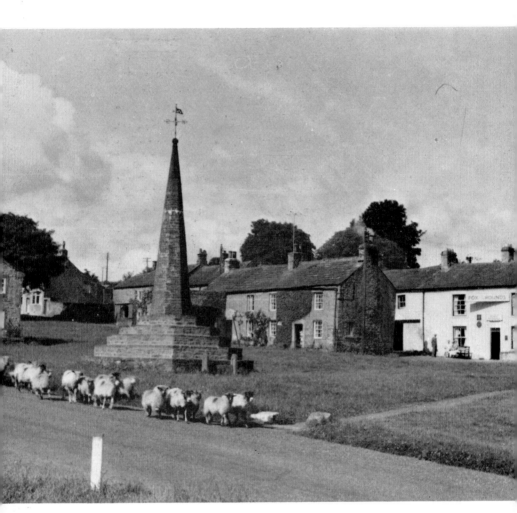

West Burton and the stocks

Russell his life as the ship to which he was later posted was torpedoed off the Isle of Wight and he was drowned.

In 1917, the *Macedonia* returned to England and Will was assigned to shore duties. Immediately after going on leave he travelled to Aysgarth, where his marriage with Gerty took place in the parish church on May 5th. Their brief honeymoon of five days was spent at Windermere. After this he was posted to Dover, where they found rooms three miles out of the town and had to have "passports" in order to get in and out of Dover. His work consisted of the usual routines of sick parades, inspections and form filling, interspersed with the occasional reception and treatment of casualties brought in from trawlers which had encountered U-boats. He did not have a great deal to do and spent much of his day studying for his M.D.

One day a great explosion rocked the town. A ship named the *Glatton* had blown up in the harbour. There were grim scenes as men fought their way up from the engine room, many of them with their clothes blasted off and suffering from extensive burns. The whole of Dover was in danger as the *Glatton* blazed, for a few yards away lay a group of ammunition ships. Will, with other naval doctors, was soon on the scene, and as he bent over the victims on the quayside giving them injections of morphia, the ammunition ships were unmoored and slowly towed out to sea. The *Glatton* was then torpedoed and sunk to avoid further danger to nearby ships, and the roads out of Dover were closed. Will could not get home and Gerty spent an anxious night as wild rumours of immense damage were circulating.

On April 23rd, 1918, the daring attempt was made by the navy to close the German submarine base at Zeebrugge with blockships. The attempt was a success but there were many casualties. Will helped to tend the five or six hundred wounded who were brought back to Dover.

The great difficulties under which the wounded were evacuated from Zeebrugge were described by a friend of Will's, Surgeon Commander James McCutcheon, who was on board the *Vindictive*.

"... The ship arrived alongside the Mole about midnight and the storming parties of seamen and marines landed immediately, followed by Surgeon Clegg and his stretcher parties. At this period, the after dressing station rapidly filled, and wardroom, cabins and Captain's quarters were successively occupied. The difficulties of landing the storming troops and embarking the wounded were aggravated by the fact that by the time the ship arrived alongside only two out of the eighteen brows (gangways) were serviceable, as the result of shell fire. The swell which had been increasing during the hour previous to arrival became considerable, and the grapnels failing to hold the ship securely alongside, the *Daffodil* performed this duty by pushing *Vindictive*'s quarter. This resulted in a succession of bumps and jars, which added to the difficulties of attending the wounded. Despite these difficulties, the transport of the wounded from the Mole to the ship was very rapid. Owing to lack of time, however, some of the cases had to be carried on board instead of being brought on the Neil-Robertson stretchers, others even being slid down the brows, the Chaplain superintending this operation from the top of the parapet. Throughout the time *Vindictive* was alongside the Mole, cases were arriving in such numbers as to make anything more than first-aid impossible in the majority of cases. Some of the cases were in great pain, and it was found that a mask sprinkled with chloroform and ether and laid on the face was welcomed by the patients while the morphia was taking effect. At one time it was found that the rate at which cases were arriving was more than the dressers could cope with, and those of the stretcher parties proficient in first-aid tended to become dressers, thereby abandoning their duties as stretcher bearers.

". . . At 1.15 a.m. *Vindictive* left the Mole and from then till berthed alongside the disembarkation pier at Dover, the medical staff was fully occupied in attending to the needs of the wounded. No attempt was made to do any operative work, as in my opinion it was out of the question. I considered it of far greater value to render advanced first-aid, counteract shock by warmth and morphia and, in fact, save the lives of serious cases till they could be dealt with at one sitting in a well-equipped hospital, where I knew they would be in a few hours' time.

During passage, tourniquets were readjusted and the outer dressings of wounds were replaced. Cases which were not under the influence of the first injection of morphia were given a second. In almost every instance where morphia had been given hypodermically, vomiting ensued when fluids were given by the mouth, but with no ill effect. Cases suffering badly from loss of blood were given saline infusions".*

With his brother Medical Officers, Will did what he could to ease the sufferings of the wounded as they lay in a shed in a railway siding at the docks awaiting transfer to the hospital train, but many were past all help and others died before they could reach Chatham hospital. It was an experience of the horrors of war which Will would never forget.

Towards the end of 1918, pestilence, the historical sequel of war broke out. The pandemic of virulent influenza which then began killed approximately nine million people throughout the world, which exceeded by far the total casualties of the war.

Will had two houses adapted as extra sick bays. Men were stricken in their billets and he had to go round with stretcher bearers and have them carried out and taken to the emergency hospital. In many instances he knew the man he was helping was doomed as his face had turned the heliotrope hue which was soon recognised as a fatal sign.

About this time Will and Gerty moved into a furnished house on the outskirts of Dover and here their first and only child, Patience, was born.

While stationed at Dover, Will took a correspondence course and sat for the M.D. examination in the summer of 1918. He was so certain that he had failed that he never went to look at the examination results when they were posted up at South Kensington. However, he had passed and so was no longer a 'doctor' merely in the eyes of the public but was entitled to that designation on the highest academic authority.

At about this time he published his first medical paper in the Royal Naval Medical Journal[1] on the subject of Vincent's disease. This was

* Journal of the Royal Naval Medical Service, January 1919

a thorough workmanlike article. He described the frequency of the condition in the Navy, the differential diagnosis from pyorrhoea alveolaris, syphilis and diphtheria, the bacteriology, the symptoms and signs illustrated by case histories, and the treatment. He noted that it was barely alluded to in the ordinary textbooks of medicine and that patients ran the risk of having all their teeth extracted under the mistaken diagnosis of pyorrhoea if it were not recognised. Later on when he first published descriptions of catarrhal jaundice, Bornholm disease, and Farmer's Lung he was to comment again on the lack of attention given to these conditions in the text books of the time.

On 20th January, 1919 he was demobilised.

The feelings experienced by Will on demobilisation were well described in an article which appeared about that time by another "temporary surgeon lieutenant".*

"After the receipt of the Demobilisation Order there is a feeling of bewilderment; the days of the present life come to a close and the threads of the old life have to be taken up again. Many of us whilst up in the Grand Fleet have toasted the day when we should return to our former "shore" billets; now that day has come and rosy visions we painted of our previous occupations seem to have faded somewhat.

"To a mouldy crowd in a wardroom it has seemed good to describe glowingly the advantages of a public service, advantages which included a motor car and gay tours through country byeways. But the description implied that the weather ashore was always fine. The prospect of those same country lanes heavy with mud, a nasty drizzle buffeting the face, and the car slithering drunkenly from side to side, is not now so alluring. Yet shore life has many compensations, but it also has many disadvantages and a narrowness of outlook often exists ashore which is not so frequently encountered at sea.

"Those were good days, jolly times, never perhaps to come back again. At first Naval discipline worried many of us, though even that we feel to have been beneficial and we return to our previous

* "A Temporary Surgeon-lieutenant", "Demobilised", Journal of the Royal Naval Medical Service, 1919, 5, 317

appointments somewhat sadly but with broader views – wiser men; sadly, because of the cheery messmates we now leave and the happy times we have spent with them; with broader views, since he who mixes with those that go down to the sea in ships mixes with men; and the wiser for our new knowledge."

Perhaps Will had less cause to regret the "jolly times" afloat. He could now look forward to a settled life with his wife and baby daughter. Within a fortnight of demobilisation he had returned to Aysgarth and had become a country doctor again.

7

THE NINETEEN-TWENTIES

DUNBAR WAS DELIGHTED to welcome his partner back. On the first day Will was called to a confinement. It was more than four years since he had done any midwifery and he soon realised how out of practice he had become in this branch of the art in which he had previously thought he had special skill. The unborn baby was head down all right, but faced forwards instead of the normal backwards. The labour dragged on and finally Will sent for Dunbar. He was greatly relieved when he heard Dunbar's motor cycle pull up outside.

While Will had been away, two sons had been born to the Dunbars, Dean and John, and a daughter, Ursula, arrived in 1920. The two families now began one of those happy experiences where two generations develop together in close friendship, helping each other and sharing each other's joys and sorrows and everyday experiences.

There was no house for the Pickles when they returned, and they settled into the Palmer Flatt, one of the two Aysgarth Inns. Here they stayed until they found rooms in the village, while the baby Patience and her nurse lived at the Post Office across the road. Then they moved to a picturesque little house in the village with no bath and an outside privy, and here they stayed for a year before moving into a house two doors below the Dunbars. Will was sick of these makeshift arrangements and decided to build a home of his own. It was not easy to buy a suitable piece of land. The farmers and land-owners seemed to regard the land as an extension of their own personalities and were reluctant to part with any of it. At last Will managed to buy for £200 a two acre field called Town Ends which lay on the left of the Aysgarth–Leyburn road, about a quarter of a mile outside the village. Here he built a comfortable four-bedroomed bungalow. Every day he would walk over to see how the house was progressing, and would explain to the three-year-old Patience who clutched his hand that these holes in the ground and the piles of bricks that lay around were to be their home. They moved in to Town Ends in April 1922. Will and Gerty lived here for over thirty years. A tennis court was laid down and became a source of continued pleasure, the beech hedges became established and the saplings they planted when they moved in became tall trees. In later years this bungalow became something of a medical Mecca for epidemiologists from all over the world.

Will and Dunbar soon resumed the routine they had followed before the war. Will was an early riser, more punctual than Dunbar and more methodical. Dunbar, in Will's absence, had developed the habit of coming to the surgery later in the morning and waiting about until 11 a.m. for occasional patients before setting off on his rounds. After Will's return, he found himself attending promptly at half-past eight while Will made out the visiting lists. Both doctors were energetic, and under Will's guidance again organised the practice so that one of them was available every day in every village. The country people had never had such a reliable service. They appreciated it and the practice grew.

In each village there was a "port of call", normally the Post Office, where patients could leave messages asking for the doctor to call or requesting another bottle of the same medicine as before. Here one of the two doctors called each day, noted the messages and left the mixtures and ointments asked for the previous day. The reason for selecting the Post Office was that they could ask whether anyone had been in to telegraph for the doctor. If a message could be intercepted in this way, it might save the annoyance of arriving back at the surgery only to find an urgent message calling the doctor out to the village he had already passed through. This system has stood the test of time and continues the same today. A small sum is paid to the postmaster annually for the slight trouble involved and he may indeed get extra custom at the shop, which is usually also part of the Post Office, as a result of people coming in to collect medicine or to leave a message.

After the war Will and Dunbar continued for a little while to use horses for some of their visits. Sometimes when their own horses were tired after the long day's round and a man arrived on horseback in the evening from high up on Walden with an urgent message, Will or Dunbar would ride back on the man's horse and tell him to wait at the surgery. Having examined the patient and made a diagnosis the doctor would ride back on the same horse and make up some medicine which the man would then take back. The whole process would take about five hours and although the horse might feel hard done by after doing the journey four times, the service had been provided and the system worked.

They kept the horses on five acres of land which they rented, but they came to rely more and more on the Ariel motor bikes and a Bradbury motor bike and side car. One year the haystack consisting of the horses' winter feed and the Dutch barn caught fire and it was found that Dunbar had forgotten to pay the insurance premium. As a consequence they sold the horses and bought a Ford Model T for £250. There were no petrol stations and they bought drums of petrol from a public house in Redmire. A self-taught mechanic in West Burton could carry out most repairs. Gerty learned to drive and to grease and oil the car and would often act as chauffeur to Will on his rounds.

Apart from improvements in transport and the gradual introduction of the telephone, the resources of the general practitioner after the 1914–18 war were not very different from those employed by John Pickles in his Leeds practice. The drugs available to Will and Dunbar in the early 1920s were much the same. *Mist. expect.*, *Mist. Scillae*, Guy's pill, arsenic, *Pot.Iod.*, bromides and alkaline mixtures were the standbys and, of course, morphia, perhaps the most useful drug of all. Will mused many years later, "When I think what I did, even as a student, prescribing ⅓ grain morphia for nearly all belly pains . . ." There was now a greater willingness to undertake surgical procedures. The partners owned a Clover's apparatus for giving ether and while Dunbar gave the anaesthetic, Will would carry out minor surgical procedures, for example, letting out the pus from an empyema and inserting a piece of boiled stethoscope tubing between the ribs as a drain. On one occasion, they diagnosed a perforated gastric ulcer. They could not obtain the services of Joe Dobson, the surgeon at Leeds, and finally persuaded Dr. Pearson of Darlington to come. They moved the kitchen table up to the bedroom and while Dunbar gave the anaesthetic, Dr. Pearson closed up the offending hole in the stomach.

By the end of the 1920s they had abandoned the practice of sending for a surgeon to come and operate in the villages, and instead the patient was sent by car or on a stretcher in the guard's van of the train to Leeds or Darlington.

Dunbar was intensely interested in the Wensleydale dialect and would come back from a round full of joy if he had collected a new word or expression. Each day they used to go over the list of visits together, thrashing out a knotty point and exchanging experiences. One day they were discussing death-beds and were agreed how rarely the fear of dying was shown, even by those who, when in full health, had a great dread of death. One of their patients, a young man who was dying of "galloping consumption" had treated the matter with extraordinary levity. The day he died he said to Will, "Well this is the end of a perfect day."

But like most doctors they hedged if patients who were dying asked if they were going to die. "Why dammit," Dunbar would say, "it's all they've got left, a bit of hope."

Dunbar had a dry sense of humour. On one occasion he was giving a lift to a very inquisitive patient who wanted to know the ailment of everyone he visited. He came out of one house with a brown paper parcel which he handed to her. "What have you brought now?" she said. "Oh," said Dean, "it's a dead baby," and she promptly dropped it. "Whatever are you doing with that?" she asked. "I'm taking it to Dr. Pickles for him to do a post mortem on and then he'll bury it."

"Why can't people bury their own babies?" said the horrified lady and then, "Oh, it does smell!"

The husband of the patient Dunbar had visited knew Will's partiality to a hare, but it being a "hunting country" he didn't want everyone to know he was sending him one. In the end Dunbar had to tell the inquisitive lady, as he feared that otherwise the fate of the "dead baby" would be circulated all over the dale.

Many of the old people whom Will attended when he first came
to the dale had been treated by his predecessors Willis, Routh and
Baker. One character, Will Mason, who lived at Woodhall, used
to go across the stepping stones over the river to the Victoria Arms
at Worton for his beer every night. His family would get worried
when he was later than usual, as he was given to stopping by the
wayside to pray when he had a "skinful". They thought he might
fall in the river. One night his son found him kneeling on one of the
stones in the middle of the swirling river where he had come to rest
on his way home from the pub. "God seave me bloody sowl," he
was wailing to the night, "God seave me bloody sowl." However,
despite his rather intemperate habits Will Mason lived till the age of
ninety-two. In his seventies he nearly died of pneumonia and at the
height of the illness his relatives suggested that a specialist should be
sent for. "Nay," said Will Mason, "if me own doctors say 'ee 'ave
to go, I'm ready and no specialist will change my opinion, but I
rayther think they'll mend me."

As trusted country doctors, Will and Dunbar naturally got to
know many of the most intimate details of their patients' lives.
Indeed this was one of the reasons why Will was later on able to
study the transmission of infectious disease so successfully. In their
early days they found that on the smaller farms some parents tried to
keep their sons at home as a source of cheap labour and their
daughters unmarried, for domestic help. Illegitimacy was not
common, but pre-marital relations followed by marriage were. In
Will's view these saved a number of unhappy childless marriages.
If a girl became pregnant her lover nearly always rose to his obligations and married her. Will did not uphold those parents who
sought to spoil the young people's love affairs often for selfish
financial reasons, and he and Dunbar sometimes rejoiced when a baby
in the offing forced their hands.

When Will returned to Aysgarth after the war, the dispensing
was done by an untrained man named Benjamin Lambert. This was
before the days when dispensers were highly trained people as they
are today. Ben had learned his trade by watching the doctors making
up the medicines. He had been taken on by Hime and was paid
ten shillings a week plus board.

Their other man was Matt Sayer. The services of both men were dispensed with in 1922 for reasons of economy. Will and Dunbar then made up their own medicines.

In 1924 there was another serious influenza epidemic. At the peak Will and Dunbar had to visit as many as a hundred homes a day, scattered up and down the dale, and see two or three times that number of patients. At such times they cursed the *malades imaginaires* in the practice. One such lady who thought she was not receiving enough care paid them an unconscious tribute when she said, "You've got to be a panel patient in Aysgarth to get proper attention."

In one such epidemic Dunbar went off sick and a locum was engaged who also retired to bed after three days. Gerty, who had picked up the rudiments of dispensing, came to the rescue washing used bottles and filling up a clothes basket with supplies of the appropriate remedy each morning for Will to take on the round. So great was the demand that they soon ran out of bottles and the villages had to be scoured for empty ones.

One of the reasons for the almost inevitable dispensing of a bottle of medicine was that it was sometimes very hard to collect a fee from the patient subsequently without this tangible evidence of a service given.

Even today if a doctor goes to a patient with influenza and says, "Stay in bed, and you will be all right in three or four days," he is unlikely to be thought of so highly as the doctor who says "Stay in bed for three or four days and take this bottle of medicine." Although both patients are equally likely to recover, the second will attribute his recovery to the medicine the doctor prescribed, while the first will probably take some remedy of his own or a friend's and attribute the cure to that. Very few patients can accept the fact that the great majority of illnesses get better whether any treatment is given or not, and this simple fact lies behind the success of all who set themselves up as healers, qualified or otherwise.

The bottles of medicine in the Aysgarth practice are no longer wrapped as neatly as they used to be and sealed with red sealing wax. The "bottle" has indeed lost caste in the face of the potent substances that have largely replaced it; the injection or the multi-coloured capsules.

Apart from Matt Sayer and Ben Lambert, the practice had the valuable accounting services of Ralph Blades. He was a remarkable man who had largely educated himself, for he had left the village school at the age of eleven. He wrote a beautiful copperplate hand, and mastered the art of keeping the books. He was also part-time sanitary inspector to the district and helped Will with his epidemiological enquiries. These accomplishments he practised as a sideline to farming and he worked in turn for Baker, Hime, and Dunbar and Will. He continued in this office until his death in 1938 at the age of seventy-nine. One of his jobs was to go up and down the dale collecting the debts, and he knew very accurately what the financial position of the practice was at any time. If Dunbar and Will decided they wanted a new motor bike, he would amost invariably counsel them against it, saying: "Now you *can't* afford it." He also got to know which patients could afford to pay their debts in full and in which cases justice should be tempered with mercy. Ralph was a just man but some of the unpopularity of the debt collector inevitably fell upon him. It is said that when he was spotted coming across the fields up to Castle Bolton, the whole population of that tiny village would unaccountably disappear into the fields, for if once Ralph got his foot in the door, he wouldn't leave without a shilling or at least sixpence towards the doctor's bill. Although in life some of the villagers may have feared his attentions, they often relied on his services in death. He was named by many in their wills as executor, so much did they admire his business acumen and respect his integrity. He was an ardent Liberal and was therefore distrusted by the Wensleydale gentry although they grudgingly acknowledged his ability. Liberals and poachers were equally detested by the gentry in those days and many a prospective tenant found it advisable to keep his politics to himself.

At first, Will quite enjoyed the business side of the practice, and as the finances improved he knew he was making that part of general practice a success. Later, he began to find the financial side of medicine more and more distasteful and one of the reasons why he strongly supported the National Health Service when it came in 1948, was that it had "taken medicine out of the market place".

In addition to the panel and private patients they had "club patients" who belonged to the Oddfellows Friendly Society and who paid five shillings, and eventually a pound, a year. Those not covered by the panel or "the club" were charged 3s 6d to 5s a visit. Poor people who were not covered by the club or panel and who couldn't afford the doctors' modest fees, would often not send for him as they were independent people. Those who were on poor relief could obtain free advice and treatment from Dunbar, and later Will, in their capacity as "the parish doctor".

In 1925 Ralph Blade's daughter Madge became dispenser to the practice and occupied a singularly important place in it for more than forty years. She was born at the Mill farm in 1890, and being highly intelligent and possessing a father who was blessed with a love of learning, and high principles, Madge developed her talents to the full. In the First World War she nursed as a V.A.D. in a Leeds hospital, and would have dearly liked to continue nursing as a career. After the war however, family reasons compelled her to return to Aysgarth. Her desire to lead a useful and practical life was satisfied, at least to some extent, when she became dispenser to the practice.

Will was very thorough in training her, and in addition to teaching her meticulously about the nature of the remedies to be prescribed and their measurement, he took great trouble in showing her how to put the pleat in the white paper wrapper round the bottle and to apply sealing wax neatly. She gradually assumed other duties besides dispensing. She would get out the panel cards on which the doctors recorded consultations, diagnoses and treatment, and later when the telephone was installed she mastered the little telephone exchange that was set up in the dispensary. This was quite a complicated arrangement as there were connections with Dr. Pickles' house, with the other partners' house, with Madge's house and with the George and Dragon, where the locums always stayed. One of the first duties of a new locum was to master this instrument, and he often ended by just learning how to telephone Madge. Having pushed the right lever up and held another down, while turning the handle at the side, he breathed a sigh of relief as the flicker went down and Madge's voice was heard speaking from her house down in the field a hundred yards away. Yes, she would come up and get through to the hospital at Northallerton, or she would telephone the ambulance, or she would inform the locum that the adrenalin was on the right-hand side of the third shelf down. Whatever the question she was never at a loss. Like the computer she could store a mass of information, but unlike it, she could retrieve it flavoured with dry Yorkshire wit.

When her father died in 1938, she also took on the task of keeping the accounts and collecting unpaid fees. She walked, or took a bus where possible, up and down the dale as she could never master the bicycle. She acquired in this way a most intimate knowledge of where the three thousand patients lived, their histories, their characters and their family relationships. This is no mean task in isolated villages where almost the whole community appears to be kith and kin. Some family names such as Metcalfe recur over and over again and it is recorded that when Sir Christopher Metcalfe was made High Sheriff of Yorkshire in 1556 he attended the judges at York accompanied by three hundred of his kinsmen riding white horses. The Metcalfes owned Nappa Hall, a fine old fortified manor house built in 1450–9 by Thomas Metcalfe. Today, it has reverted to the more simple status of an ordinary farm, but a Metcalfe still lives there.

In addition to their general duties, Dunbar and Will looked after tuberculous patients in the private Wensleydale Sanatorium owned by an enterprising character named Joseph Smith with a side line in horse breeding. They called there on alternate days after their evening meal and would enjoy a glass of wine with the proprietor after seeing the patients.

The office of part-time Medical Officer of Health for Aysgarth Rural District was held in turn by Baker, Hime and Dunbar, and after Dunbar died in 1935, by Will. The salary paid to the doctor responsible for safeguarding the health of this district was £60 a year plus £20 travelling expenses.

This modest appointment had its amusing side. On one occasion an enquiry was being held into the public health risks entailed by the proximity of a milking shed to the new sewage works and the following exchange took place:

Magistrate: "You are a practical farmer I believe, McAllen. If you

were farming this land would you remove your milking
shed from the proximity of the sewage works?"

Farmer: "Nay, I'd remove t'sewage works".

Two other part-time medical appointments were held by the
doctors in the Aysgarth practice – that of District Medical Officer,
and that of medical officer to the "workhouse" at Bainbridge. For
the former, a salary of £50 a year was paid in 1947 and for the latter
£40. The appointment of District Medical Officer finally came to
an end with the passing of the National Health Service Act in 1948.
With the abolition of pauperism and the provision of a free medical
service for all, this stop-gap service designed to mitigate one of the
harsher results of poverty ceased to be required. Will continued,
however, to look after patients in the Public Assistance Institution
which became a Welfare Home after 1948.

Under Will and Dunbar the size of the practice increased. People
who lived in Bainbridge who had had Hawes doctors gradually
transferred to them. At the lower end of the dale, that part of the
practice at Preston-under-Scar which had been largely won over by
Hime, was transferred to Will's brother Jack who was in practice in
Leyburn, for a small sum. In West Witton a certain number of the
population went to the much loved George Cockroft of Middleham,
but this was less convenient than Aysgarth, and most of these
ultimately transferred their allegiance to the Aysgarth doctors. Thus
the practice was defined and consolidated in the form in which it
exists to the present day. This was very valuable to Will in his
epidemiological investigations as it meant that virtually everyone
in the geographical area covered by the practice was available for
study.

There are always patients who become discontented with their
doctors and who will seek farther afield if they think there is another
doctor who may understand them better. The Aysgarth doctors,
however, would refuse to accept patients from villages outside their
area, and this custom was followed by the neighbouring doctors.
There were many advantages in this understanding. By removing
competition for patients and causes for jealousy, it helped to avoid
friction between the G.P.s in the dale and it meant that the doctor

would not be called to see perhaps a discontented and troublesome patient a long way from his centre of practice.

The early twenties were halcyon days for the two young doctors and their families. There were plenty of tennis parties arranged by themselves or by the "gentry" at the big houses. There were shooting parties on the moors, golf at Leyburn or Hawes and fishing in the Ure. Will's father-in-law, Mr. Tunstill, rented the stretch of river between the old ford and Worton, and here Will would sometimes fish or watch the sand martins swerving about over the water and darting into their nesting holes in the miniature sandy cliffs that contain this stretch of river. With Dean Dunbar he rented a rough shoot at £5 a year on Haw Bank on the road from Askrigg to Carperby. They would organise shoots in the autumn and hire a few beaters. From this shoot they would take pheasants, snipe, woodcock and rabbits. It could have been said of them at this period "And they found fat pasture and good, and the land was wide, and quiet and peaceable".*

If Will had not been an exceptional man, he might have been content to live the absorbing and relatively uncomplicated life of a country doctor, caring for his patients conscientiously and enjoying the peaceful pleasures of country life. He was now forty, established and respected. But in 1926 he came across a book which greatly influenced him. It was called *The Principles of Diagnosis and Treatment in Heart Affections*, by James Mackenzie. Mackenzie was also a general practitioner.

* I Chronicles 4, 40

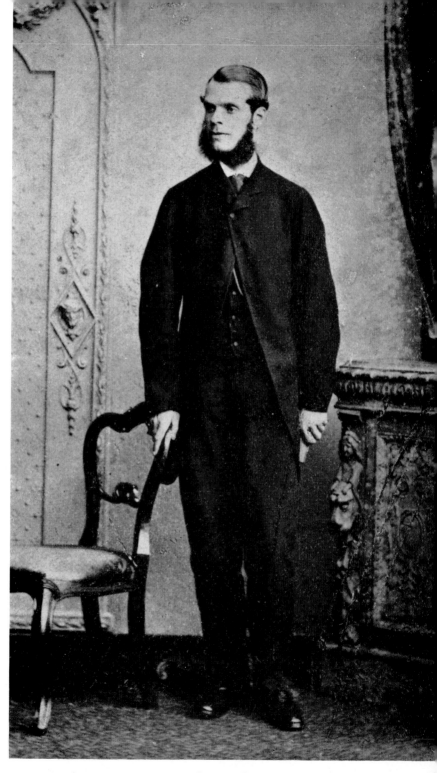

Dr. Matthew Willis aged 43

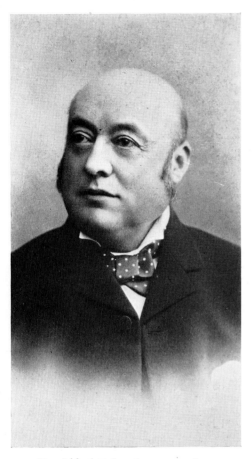 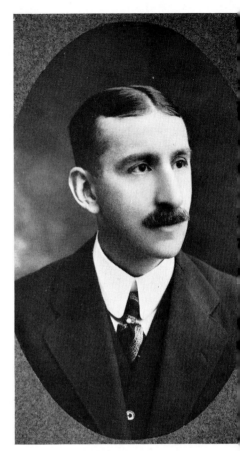

Dr. Alfred Baker *d.* 1903 aged 55   Dr. Edward Hime *d.* 1934

8

NEW HORIZONS

MACKENZIE'S BOOK* MADE a deep impression on Will. Here was a general practitioner who had begun making his original observations on the irregularities of the pulse which had made him famous, while still in general practice.

Mackenzie later became a consultant physician to the London Hospital, but he retained his interest in general practice and his conviction that the general practitioner was in a uniquely favourable position to observe disease from its earliest onset and therefore to check its development.

In his book he had written:

"The time is approaching when, in the course of nature, I must fall out of the ranks, and before doing so I wish to look back upon my medical career to see what light my experience may throw upon medical sciences. The life of a general practitioner is not considered one that can help much in the advance of medicine; it is, indeed, regarded so lightly that no steps are ever taken to train one who intends to become a general practitioner in any branch that would enable him to undertake research work. You know well that if a man aspires to research work it is to the laboratories or to the hospital wards he is sent. As a result of my experience, I take a very different view, and assert with confidence that medicine will make but halting progress, while whole fields essential to the progress of medicine will remain unexplored, until the general practitioner takes his place as an investigator. The reason for this is that he has opportunities which no other worker

* *The Principles of Diagnosis and Treatment in Heart Affections.* 1st Edn. 1916, 2nd Edn. 1923, 3rd Edn. 1926

G

possesses – opportunities which are necessary to the solution of problems essential to the advance of medicine . . ."

In order better to promote these ideas Mackenzie eventually gave up his consultant appointment in London to become the first director of the Institute for Clinical Research at St. Andrews. At the first meeting of the staff of the Institute the following resolution was passed:

"The main objects of research would be the early stages of disease, and the work would primarily consist of the detailed observations of symptoms and the keeping of careful records. Prolonged observations of cases would be carried out in order to discover the significance of early symptoms, and researches would be undertaken with a view to ascertaining the mechanism of their production".*

Mackenzie's recognition of the great opportunities for original research presented to the general practitioner was far ahead of his time, It is only recently, and largely due to the example of Will Pickles and to the efforts of the Royal College of General Practitioners, that a substantial number of general practitioners have started to undertake research in their practices.

Mackenzie's book and career proved to Will that it was possible for a general practitioner to make original and important observations, and it may not be an exaggeration to suggest that it was this book which was responsible for him setting out at the age of forty-two on the road which made him famous. In the years following the war he had felt he was drifting, but now he determined to go forward.

In 1927, in order to bring his medical knowledge up to date, he took a correspondence course in medicine arranged by a "cram" school in London. He did the required reading and diligently answered the set questions at the end of his day's work. But knowledge by post did not satisfy him. He felt he should return to the hospital atmosphere to see and hear consultants demonstrating actual cases and to learn, from the men at the top, the latest methods of diagnosis and treatment.

* R. McNair Wilson, *The Beloved Physician: Sir James Mackenzie.*

In 1929 he went for a month's refresher course to London and spent two weeks at St. John's Hospital for diseases of the skin and uro-genital system, and two weeks at the West London Hospital. The next year he went to the Edinburgh Royal Infirmary for a month. He continued to go for a month's refresher course at different hospitals every year until 1939. Dunbar, who might have resented him leaving the practice in this way, generously encouraged him. "You go, Will," he would say, "and come back and tell me what you have learned."

As part-time deputy Medical Officer of Health for the rural district of Aysgarth Will had some responsibility for the tracing and control of epidemics.

In 1928 an epidemic of jaundice started in the dale which stimulated him to start his researches on the transmission of infectious illnesses. This was the same disease which had puzzled him when he was an assistant in Bedale in 1910. Now he decided to investigate it systematically. He wrote of this decision as follows:

"Dunbar and I had always been interested in our epidemics, thinking it great fun when we could exercise Sherlock Holmes tactics and nail the culprits, but it was not until 1929 I came to the conclusion that we really should make more use of our opportunities. This was borne forcibly upon me by the presence of an epidemic of jaundice. There had been very little written about it. What interested me enormously was that my records seemed to indicate a long incubation period, much longer than any other zymotic disease, indeed up to a month and sometimes even longer."

Will had read most of the classical works on epidemiology: John Snow on cholera, William Budd on typhoid fever and Creighton's *History of Epidemics in Britain*, and he determined to become an authority on epidemics in this country. Dunbar was aware of this and was interested and helpful.

Catarrhal jaundice, as infectious hepatitis used to be called, although not usually responsible for severe epidemics in peacetime often reaches epidemic proportions in wartime.

The epidemic which Will now decided to study turned out to be unusually severe. Out of a total estimated population in Wensleydale of 5,700 there were 250 known cases of jaundice of whom Will and Dunbar attended 118. The rest were seen by other doctors from Hawes or Leyburn, or did not seek medical attention. Will was particularly interested in the apparently long incubation period which his records suggested, and he now set himself to confirm more precisely the length of this period by carefully noting in his diary the date of onset of symptoms in all cases and the dates of contacts with other known cases. He wrote to the Ministry of Health to find out what was known about the epidemiology of this disease, and an epidemiologist, Dr. W. A. Lethem, came to visit him. Together they visited houses and schools collecting epidemiological data. Gradually the pattern of infection emerged.

The first patient developing the disease in Bainbridge, for example, was found to have spent an afternoon at the house of a cousin in Aysgarth a month before. The cousins in Aysgarth had been poorly at the time of the visit and had become yellow the day after. This sort of occurrence, which Will termed "the short and only possible contact", when repeated over and over again, established the incubation period as 26 to 35 days. The fascinating detective work that lay behind these bald figures is best told in Will's own words:[10]

"The five names . . . are those of the only sufferers from jaundice in the whole district who commenced in the week September 24 to October 1. Three of these were from the village in which the fête was held on August 28, and I found, as I expected, that they had all been present. I felt sure also that I was on the track of an interesting discovery when it transpired that the other two from distant villages had this, and only this, experience in common with these three. Someone suffering from jaundice, therefore, had also probably been a visitor at the fête. I tried various sources, and at last, after a long search, I discovered the culprit where I least expected, almost on my own doorstep.

"This was a young girl (B) whom I had actually seen in bed on the very morning of the fête and who I never dreamt would be able to get up that day. I have no doubt she exercised considerable skill and elusiveness at the entertainment, for I was also among the throng and did not know of her presence. This girl had as a friend another girl of 16 (E) who lived in a distant village, and these two young girls spent the afternoon together, with the result that E herself commenced with the disease on October 1, and infected four others in this village. She was employed as a maid, and she infected her employer's small son, this boy's friend, and her own great-aunt, who lived in the village. The infection in all these was easy to explain, but in the fourth (M), a rather pathetic little fellow of middle age, it was not so clear. At last I tackled his sister, who gave him away quite shamelessly. Studies in epidemiology sometimes reveal romances. "Oh yes," she said, "he's very fond of E. He often goes in at the back door in the evenings, and helps her to wash up." The brother of M in the same house commenced on December 5, and the faithless sister, above mentioned, with poetic justice succumbed on January 4. J, who was a friend of H and E, commenced on November 4, his small brother on December 8, and this small brother's friend on January 8. Thus, to my knowledge, thirteen instances of this disease resulted from the determination of one young girl, jaundice or no jaundice, not to be deprived of what she considered her legitimate amusement."

Will first described this epidemic in an article which he sent to the British Medical Journal on New Year's Day 1930. He received the usual acknowledgement slip but after that heard nothing. After three months had passed he wrote to the editor to see if they were going to accept the article or not. The editor replied that it was too long and that the case histories were tedious. Like most authors Will found this criticism hard to swallow, and with some bitterness re-wrote the article. He was sure he knew best what should go in and what should be excluded, but rather than risk not having it published he cut it by half to about 2,000 words and it finally appeared in May, 1930.[2] He was disappointed when it seemed to make little impression on the profession. No editorial comment was devoted to his report but he did receive a number of letters from other G.P.s. However, a year later Sir William Willcox, physician to St. Mary's Hospital, London, referred to it in his Lumleian lecture to the Royal College of Physicians in 1931 as follows: "An interesting account of a recent

epidemic (of infectious hepatitis) in Yorkshire was published by
Pickles."

Will had discovered after finishing his study that two other
investigators* had previously published a similar report on an
epidemic of catarrhal jaundice and had given a rather wider range of
incubation times, 20 to 40 days. At about the same time Dr. Alison
Glover, then Chief Medical Officer at the Ministry of Education,
was maintaining records of epidemics at residential schools and held
the opinion that epidemic jaundice had a shorter incubation period
than that assigned to it by Will. Will wrote to Glover and asked if
he could come down and discuss the problem with him. He accord-
ingly visited Glover at the Ministry of Education. "After a long
interview in which I vainly tried to convince him of the error of his
ways, we got down to brass tacks," wrote Will. "I told him I thought
the country doctor could supply much information, but did not
know quite how to keep records. He showed me the charts that were
being kept in certain boarding schools in a Medical Research Council
investigation he was conducting and we both saw how readily these
could be adapted for a self-contained country practice." A firm
friendship developed between Will and Alison Glover.

There is no doubt that Will's warm and friendly nature opened
many doors to him. He was always willing to travel long distances
and take infinite trouble to learn from someone whom he thought
could help him. Later on he would do the same for visitors to
Aysgarth and impart, even to the most junior doctor or medical
student, his knowledge of epidemics gained from his own first hand
experience. From Alison Glover he got the idea of keeping time
charts of all his cases of infectious disease. Each disease was given a
symbol. For example a case of measles was represented as a blue
square and a case of influenza as a red one, and marked in on the day
when the symptoms started (see chart facing p. 114).

Patience, then aged thirteen, started keeping these charts for her
father in 1931. Later on Gerty undertook the rather laborious task of
keeping them up to date, and carried it on with meticulous care for
more than twenty years.

* W. E. Booth and C. C. Okell, "Epidemic Catarrhal Jaundice", Public Health
1928, 41, 237

Will was not fond of driving, and when Patience left school at seventeen she obtained a driving licence and chauffeured her father on his rounds. By getting to know all the dales folk and keeping notes for Will she was able to relieve him of some of the routine work involved in a general practice and to free some of his time for his epidemiological work.

Will's meetings with Alison Glover set him firmly on the road as a practical epidemiologist. In November 1931 an outbreak of Sonne dysentery started in the dale and Will described the outbreak in a short article in the Lancet[3]:

"The next cases to be seen were on January 4th of this year, when a message was sent from a farm, where a truly deplorable condition obtained. A mother and four young children were prostrate in two beds in one room. The stench was almost intolerable, and the poor victims were lying helpless in their evacuations. One little boy had had a fit, and two others had bled profusely enough to cause alarm.

"The epidemic in none of the villages was of a fulminating nature suggesting water contamination. The first case in every village was known, and there was a gradual rise and a gradual fall in the number of cases, which pointed strongly to a spread of the disease by personal contact alone. The conveyers of the disease from village to village were identified, although all attempts to discover where the disease came from in the first instance have failed.

"The last village to be attacked was naturally investigated more completely, 44 cases occurring out of a population of 110. By ill chance the mother of the largest family in the village entertained a sufferer from one of the other villages to tea on January 29. On the 31st her first symptoms appeared, and between February 7 and 20 her husband and her nine children were successively attacked."

Specimens of faeces from six of the victims were obtained and sent off to the Ministry of Health. All were found to contain the Sonne dysentery bacillus.

The following year another disease not clearly recognised

previously in Great Britain dramatically claimed Will's attention.
He described the circumstances thus:

"In the early morning of a bright July day in 1933 I was roused
from my bed by a young farmer who, I knew, was of a placid
disposition and gifted with common sense, but who on this
occasion was thoroughly alarmed. He asked if I would come to
one of his small boys who had been taken seriously ill. This boy,
aged 2½ years, had been quite well and lively whilst being dressed,
but was then attacked suddenly with pain in the upper abdomen,
sweated profusely, and was thought by his mother to have had a
fit. When I saw him the pain was not so acute, but he was limp and
deadly pale and looked extremely ill. He was taking short shallow
breaths, which were obviously causing him discomfort, but at this
stage his temperature was only 98°F. Later in the morning my
partner saw him in a return of the acute pain, and suggested that
the trouble was a painful spasm of the diaphragm. This was a very
acute clinical observation which helped us materially in the final
decision on the identity of the disease. We saw him together at
3 p.m. and again the picture was changed. His face was flushed,
his temperature was 101°, and his respirations were definitely 60
per minute. The respiration rate, we knew, was most unusually
high, and neither of us could remember counting such a rate,
except in pneumonia patients who were obviously not going to
recover.

"The boy was lying in a dazed condition, taking no notice of
what we were doing as we examined him, his alae nasi were
working, he had an expiratory grunt and a short cough.

"At this point we felt we were on firmer ground and were
justified in suggesting to the parents that the child was commencing
with acute pneumonia, although there were no physical signs of
this disease . . . In the evening he seemed slightly better, which
added somewhat to our difficulties if at the same time it added to
our peace of mind. His temperature had come down to 100°, he
appeared to have lost his respiratory distress, and he had no pain.
The next morning it was obvious we were dealing with a strange
disorder. The little rascal, standing on the window-sill and

thumping on the pane, greeted me smilingly, but, I thought, derisively, as I walked up the garden path. I examined him carefully and could find nothing to account for the happenings of the previous day. I told his mother, without beating about the bush, that I had not the slightest idea what had been the matter with her child, but that he was quite well again and that she need not worry any more about him. This was an extremely rash remark, as I was to learn to my cost later, for the next morning I found the boy in very much the same condition as he was on the first day of the illness, and he had several hours of similar distressing symptoms, with the addition of pain in the back, which prevented him from raising himself in the bed. The next day he had a 'bad cold in the head' and his evening temperature was 99·8°, but he soon afterwards completely recovered.

"The family consisted of father and mother and three little boys in addition to the first victim, and the boon companions of the boys were three little girls who lived on the other side of the road. Two of these were bending over the sufferer's couch with interest and solicitude depicted on their features on the very first day of his illness. I told the mother that these young women would be better to remain in their own home until we had decided what was the matter with her own child and they were packed off. I little thought that the damage had already been done . . . Two of the brothers were attacked on the second and third days respectively of the first boy's illness, and the two little girls on the fourth day.

"We were, therefore, dealing with a small epidemic of infectious disease of very definite syndrome, but of which our textbooks told us nothing."

The outbreak was traced to a little girl from York who had come to the farm of the first victim for a "day's treat" four days before the little boy became ill. This young visitor had spent the day doubled up on the sofa sobbing with pain and had not enjoyed her treat at all.

Will recalled that he had received, about a year before, a reprint of an article by a Danish general practitioner, Dr. E. Sylvest. The English summary of this article indicated that Sylvest had described in the Danish island of Bornholm a condition similar to that now occurring in Wensleydale.

Will sent an account of his cases to the editor of the British Medical Journal asking the editor to return it if he found it devoid of interest. In reply he received the proofs of the article and it was published in the B.M.J. on November 4th, 1933 under the title "Bornholm Disease": Account of a Yorkshire Outbreak".[4] In the article he acknowledged the help he had received from Sylvest's article and also quoted earlier descriptions of what was apparently the same disease by other authors who had called it "devil's grip" on account of the very severe pain in the chest or back which the sufferers experience, or epidemic pleurisy.

Will Pickles confirmed the occurrence of the disease in Great Britain, and his vivid and careful account of its symptoms served to bring the disease into the minds of other doctors when confronted with a patient with these symptoms. This must have prevented a good many wrong diagnoses and probably a good many healthy appendices from being taken out unnecessarily.

Sylvest had also written a paper on epidemic jaundice, and he and Will had exchanged reprints of their articles.

Will kept notes of infectious diseases for over a quarter of a century. At times it was not easy, as epidemics of influenza, for example, not only greatly increased the load of work but often affected the doctors themselves, as happened in the influenza epidemic of 1937. Charting of the epidemics at these times was the last straw, but every night they were written up and the record continued.

One of the villages, West Burton, escaped lightly in the 1937 epidemic of influenza, but in 1933, when there had been a full-scale epidemic in the country at large, West Burton had suffered badly. On the earlier occasion the schoolmistress, after a holiday at Scarborough, had managed to struggle to school for one brief morning session and caused the disease in seventy-eight victims. Will mentioned this to Professor, later Sir, McFarlane Burnet of Melbourne, who visited him in 1946, and he took Will's data back to Australia with him. From this it was concluded that there is a definite immunity from a given strain of influenza in a village population which lasts for about four years, but which fades altogether in seven.

In addition to his annual refresher course Will began to take his family farther afield on their summer holidays. Soon after their return from one of these holidays in September 1934 there was a call for Dunbar to go to a lonely hamlet high above Bainbridge. To Will's surprise, Dunbar said he didn't think he could manage the walk up to the farm from the road as he had a painful leg. Will did the visit and the next day Dunbar couldn't turn out at all owing to a painful swelling of his leg. Thrombosis of a vein in the lowest part of the leg was diagnosed. Dunbar had to go to bed and a locum was obtained. Later he had all his teeth extracted as it was thought that dental sepsis might be the cause of the trouble. After two months he was up and about and beginning to work again. One day he said to Will, "Now I feel perfectly well. You can put the night bell on to me." The next day Dunbar had a long round. He incised an abscess at Redmire and went on as usual to West Witton. Just before lunch Will received a message that Dunbar had felt faint during a consultation, had hurried out to the kitchen and vomited into the sink. Will hurried to the scene and found his partner lying unconscious on the kitchen floor breathing stertorously, his face a livid hue. A boy was sent to the Post Office to telephone for the ambulance, and the post-mistress sent him back for the money for the call. It seemed to Will a very long time before the ambulance came. Dean Dunbar died twelve hours later without regaining consciousness. Dr. Eddison of Bedale signed the death certificate and attributed the death to an embolus.

So this happy partnership was abruptly ended. Dunbar, like Willis and Baker before him, was buried in Aysgarth churchyard and the church was not large enough to accommodate the dalesfolk who came to pay their last tribute. Another plaque was set up on the wall of the church:

"Giving thanks to God for his devoted service to the dales from 1909–1934.
This tablet is placed here in memory of Dean Dunbar, M.B.B.S. Lond. by his friends."

Dean Dunbar is still remembered by the older generation in the dale, and I saw on the wall of a patient's house a photo of the Board of Guardians in 1926 showing Will and Dunbar. As I looked at it and asked what Dunbar was like, the old man commented with affection and respect, "He was blunt, you know".

Will felt the loss of Dunbar deeply. It seemed a savage stroke that he should die so unexpectedly in his prime. Will now had to engage a succession of locums until he could find someone to replace Dunbar on a more permanent footing. Some stayed only for a week or two while others stayed for months. One typical "perpetual" locum was lazy and drank to excess. He would see ten patients a day while Will managed thirty. The patients loved him, however, because he took plenty of time talking to them and listening to their troubles.

A physician at Darlington, in whom Will had great faith, told a doctor of his acquaintance, Dr. Ord, that Will was looking for a partner. As a result Ord visited the practice two or three times and Will invited him to become a partner. The new partner put a sum of money down as part of the purchase price of his share of the practice and after a further delay due to an attack of influenza he finally arrived at the end of April 1934. Ord was a good doctor and seemed determined to succeed. He and Will got on well at first but somehow the partnership did not prosper.

However, a *modus vivendi* was found, and the partnership endured until 1945. Will did not allow these difficulties to discourage him from pursuing his epidemiological enquiries.

9

GROWING REPUTATION AND "EPIDEMIOLOGY IN COUNTRY PRACTICE"

SOON AFTER HIS article on the epidemic of Bornholm disease appeared, Will read the Herter lectures given by Professor Major Greenwood on "Epidemiology, Historical and Experimental".* This prompted him to send a reprint of his article together with some of his epidemiological charts to Major Greenwood, who was then head of the Department of Epidemiology and Medical Statistics at the London School of Hygiene and Tropical Medicine. Greenwood was a great admirer of William Budd (1811–1880), the Devonshire country doctor who had in the course of his general practice worked out and described the mode of spread of typhoid fever, and on receiving Will's charts Greenwood remarked to a colleague, "This is the most outstanding happening in epidemiology in the last twenty-five years". He thought that he might have discovered in Will Pickles a successor to Budd, and invited him to visit him in London.

Greenwood was a remarkable man. Small in stature and apparently mild in disposition he could be a tiger when opposed. He was the son and grandson of East End general practitioners and himself became a G.P. in Shoreditch after he qualified. The humanitarianism with which he was imbued in consequence of his upbringing and experience in general practice is revealed in his advice to those who wished to carry out research in social medicine:

> "Do not forget there is a research laboratory greater even than the Cavendish, the streets, the homes, the factories in which common people pass their lives – there is the laboratory of him who adds to our knowledge of social medicine".

* Major Greenwood, *Epidemiology, Historical and Experimental*, O.U.P., 1932

Later on, his own "liking for sums", as he put it, led him into academic fields, and he became a distinguished medical statistician and with his successor Professor, later Sir Austin, Bradford Hill, helped to introduce many of the statistical methods now used in epidemiology and in the scientific assessment of new forms of treatment.

In December 1934 Will lunched with Greenwood and Bradford Hill at the London School of Hygiene. It was a great occasion for him. He met other doctors working at the School, and began to feel he was no longer working in isolation but had joined a distinguished company of British epidemiologists. Perhaps he would one day achieve his niche of fame with men like Graunt, Jenner, Budd, Farr and Snow: men who had looked beyond the individual sick person and had discovered that beyond the laws governing the manifestations of disease in an individual there were other natural laws amenable to investigation which determine the incidence and distribution of illness in the community. On parting, Greenwood said to him, "Now you must write a book, Pickles." With this idea implanted in his mind Will returned to the dale and soon began to write the slender volume which was to become a medical classic.

The next year he was invited to speak in London at a meeting of the Epidemiological Section of the Royal Society of Medicine. There was a good attendance, and the audience included some of the most eminent and critical epidemiologists of the time including Major Greenwood, Bradford Hill, Alison Glover and Percy Stocks. Will referred to his paper as "a crude and immature performance aided by some wall diagrams and the epidiascope". However, it apparently went down well as there were many questions and it stimulated a leading article in the British Medical Journal* which said, "We trust that when the full text of Dr. Pickles' latest paper is available, it will be widely read. We are even sanguine enough to hope that it may mark the beginning of a new era in epidemiology. If only Dr. Pickles' example were to inspire others practising in sparsely populated districts, others to whom also the facts are something more vivid than entries in a statistical daybook, progress would be certain."

* Brit. med. J. 1935, 1, 1227

In his paper Will had described how he was able to show, by examples of "the short and only possible exposure", that the incubation period of measles, from infection to onset of rash, could be as short as twelve days. He also described three cases of shingles occurring in people who had been exposed to chicken pox and the epidemic of influenza already referred to in which a teacher returning from a holiday resort with the illness had infected seventy-eight others.

In the discussion which followed Dr. J. D. Rolleston, the chairman, said that Dr. Pickles had shown what excellent epidemiological work could be done by country doctors, and Professor Greenwood described his work as "fundamental epidemiology". A member of the audience asked if Will had seen any cases of undulant fever in his practice, to which Will replied with typical modesty that there had been a case a few years previously but that he had missed the diagnosis.

Life for Will and Gerty began to expand. In the summer of 1936 they went on a cruise and visited Copenhagen in order to meet Dr. Sylvest. He was on holiday in the island of Bornholm at the time but came home and opened up his house in Copenhagen to entertain them. With Dr. Sylvest and his wife and sister they visited the Tivoli gardens and went out to dinner and a theatre. The next day Will was shown the hospitals and laboratories and he and Sylvest discussed at length their common experiences of Bornholm disease and epidemic jaundice.

Throughout this period and right up to the Second World War Will continued to attend refresher courses, usually in London, for one month in each year. In addition he developed his contacts and friendships at the London School of Hygiene and went to the meetings of the "Tea Club" where he met among others Dr. May Smith, Dr. W. R. Russell and Professor, later Sir, Wilson Jameson. Jameson was then Professor of Public Health at the School. Later he became Chief Medical Officer at the Ministry of Health. He was about Will's age, and his quiet geniality appealed to Will. Will admired the efficiency with which he ran his department at the School, and later enjoyed his friendship throughout his active and successful period at the Ministry during the Second World War

where among other achievements he succeeded in extending
diphtheria immunisation widely throughout the country. The result
was that this dreaded disease, which was killing two or three thousand
children in the United Kingdom each year before Jameson's campaign, has virtually disappeared from Great Britain. Diphtheria
inoculation had been available for some years before and had already
been widely and successfully introduced in Canada. Why we were
so slow in introducing it on a large scale here might make an
interesting historical study.

Will had become part-time Medical Officer of Health for the
Aysgarth district following Dunbar's death, and had started immun-
ising school children against diphtheria in 1936. Later he initiated a
campaign to immunise all the children in his district. There was one
small outbreak at Askrigg in 1939, introduced by evacuees at the
outbreak of the war, but after this no further cases seem to have
occurred in the district.

Soon after Will became part-time M.O.H. for his district Dr.,
later Sir, Andrew Davidson was appointed M.O.H. for the North
Riding. One of his duties was to visit the tuberculosis sanatorium at
Aysgarth of which Will was Medical Officer. Will would ask him
to lunch and he often stayed on for dinner. A warm friendship grew
up between the two men and Will would drive to Northallerton,
about twenty miles away, for quarterly meetings of the North
Riding Medical Officers of Health which Davidson arranged. Will
became secretary of this group and himself gave a short paper on
diphtheria immunisation. Later on when the threat of war was
deepening they had a discussion on "Problems of Evacuation". They
started off these meetings in the early afternoon with tea and
biscuits and after the meeting they would adjourn to the local
inn where any possible misunderstandings could be ironed out
and friendships fostered under the benign influence of Yorkshire
ale.

About this time Will was asked to lecture to the Leeds Medical
Society. He was beginning to overcome his shyness of public
speaking from which he had always suffered. His method of delivering a speech or lecture always remained the same. He wrote it out in
full in manuscript and then more or less learned it by heart. He was

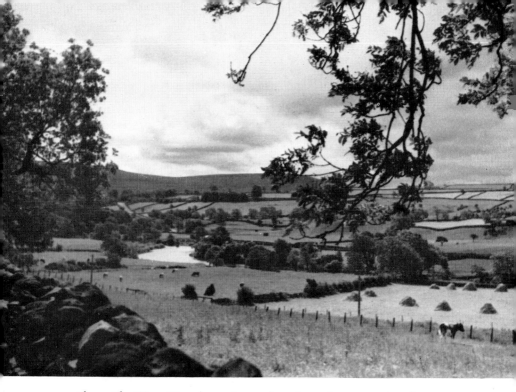

Above. The River Ure above Aysgarth. *Below*. The Aysgarth Falls

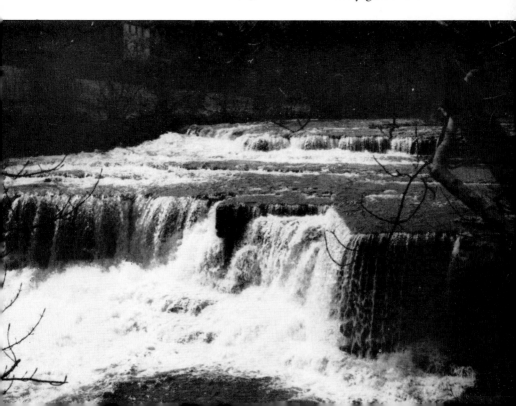

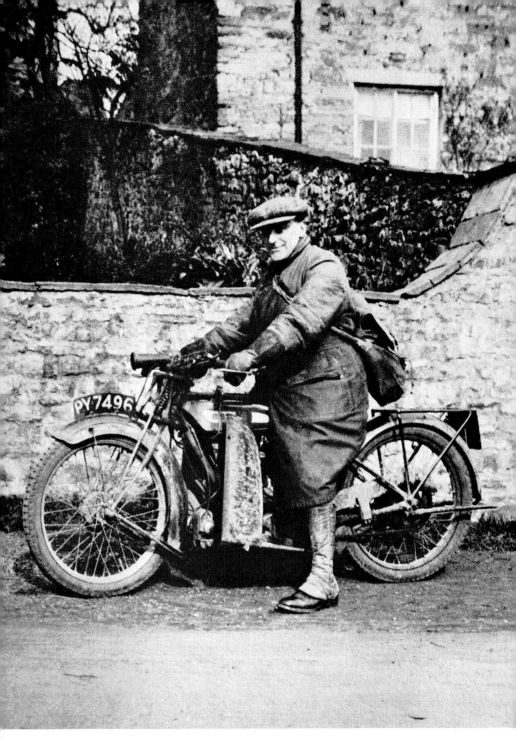

Dr. Dean Dunbar on his round

therefore able to speak without notes and having a natural and easy delivery sounded completely spontaneous. A careful listener might perhaps detect that the sentences were a little too well constructed and the choice of words a little too apt for the speech not to have been composed and well conned beforehand. He always carried a copy of his speech or lecture in his breast pocket or in a leather wallet on the desk in front of him in case his memory should let him down, but it never did.

Following Greenwood's suggestion that he should write a book on epidemiology, Will kept even more careful and complete records of all cases of infectious disease in the practice. On his rounds he jotted down in his diary the name and village of each victim and the date of onset. At home he transcribed these notes to a large stiff-backed foolscap book, a relic of his naval days. In this he grouped the cases by family and village, displaying an epidemic on a single page and giving clinical histories of typical and interesting cases. The same book was used to make notes on lectures he attended at various courses over the years. Out of this apparent disorder he was able by diligent work between tea and supper to write a medical classic. Evening surgeries in the Aysgarth practice were kept to a minimum and often there were no patients at all. But for this fact the book might never have been written. He wrote the first version in the winter of 1937 and re-wrote it in 1938. To Will's great disappointment, *Epidemiology in Country Practice* was turned down by several well-known publishers. Finally, however, it was published by John Wright of Bristol in May 1939.[10] This book established Will's reputation as an epidemiologist and ensured his place in the history of medicine. In 110 pages it contained the essence of his observations of infectious disease systematically observed and recorded over the previous ten years.

In the preface Greenwood wrote: "The old race of epidemiologists is *not* extinct. We have indeed had to wait a long time for a second Budd, but I think we have found one. I firmly believe that the epidemiology of our own country will receive a fresh impulse from discoveries made, not by experts, but by medical practitioners working patiently on the lines of Dr. Pickles".

Almost at the beginning of the book Will acknowledged his debt

H

to William Budd and appealed to his fellow country doctors to make use of their opportunities, quoting Budd as follows:

"It is obvious that the formation of just opinions on the question how diseases spread may depend less on personal ability than on the opportunities for its determination which may fall to the lot of the observer. It is equally obvious that where the question at issue is that of the propagation of disease by human intercourse, rural districts, where the population is thin, and the lines of intercourse are few and always easily traced, offer opportunities for its settlement which are not to be met with in the crowded haunts of large towns.

"The object of this book", Will continued, "is to stimulate other country doctors to keep records of epidemic disease and to put before them the unique advantages that their position gives them, to impress on those interested in epidemiology the value of the natural history method of investigation of these diseases, and to awaken some interest in the layman, whose help in these matters cannot be overestimated. I personally cannot acknowledge too gratefully the help I have received in my own investigations from my patients."

Referring to the other doctor who greatly influenced him he wrote:

"Sir James Mackenzie wrote emphatically on the advantages of general practice as a medium for research, contending that it was the family doctor who alone saw disease in its true perspective, as he had the advantage of observing early symptoms and following an illness from beginning to end."

There follows a chapter on "The Lines of Communication" which includes a description of the geology of the dale, the use of parish registers to study the epidemics of the past and the influence of holidays and outings and the grammar school on the spread of infectious disease.

He described his technique of recording the onset of symptoms of every case of infectious disease and the linking of cases by discovering the "short and only possible contact" to establish the incubation period and the period of infectiousness illustrated in the coloured charts.

The ensuing chapters deal with the epidemiology of the common fevers. In each case epidemics that occurred in the dale are described in simple and attractive English and in such a way that the reader is made to feel he is actually taking part in the tracking down of the source of some epidemic.

Separate chapters are devoted to the two diseases which Will made his particular study: epidemic jaundice and Bornholm disease. They constitute classical descriptions of the clinical epidemiological features of those two conditions.

Epidemiology in Country Practice was well received. The Lancet reviewer wrote: "Dr. Pickles may not see a dozen cases of zoster in all his years of practice; yet Dr. Pickles' single record is worth more to epidemiology than the thousands of cases which have been casually noted in London in the past ten years . . . the whole book should be read by every country doctor."

In Public Health, the reviewer noted: "If, as Tolstoy says, labour is the joyful business of life, then Dr. Pickles is indeed a fortunate man, for in this book he shows how epidemiology, always a fascinating subject, can be such an inspiration to a busy practitioner as to enable him to prove that it is the busiest persons who have time for everything, to collect an amazing amount of detailed facts and to make the pursuit of knowledge a joy itself and something infinitely more than a means to an end."

He received many letters from old friends about the book. Alison Glover wrote: "Hearty congratulations on the new classic. It is a delightful book with the deceptive simplicity of real art. I am very proud to have your kind mention and I shall be remembered by it when all my own works are long forgotten. It will live." Ejnar Sylvest from Copenhagen wrote: "Very many thanks for your beautiful and most interesting book which I read with great pleasure. You are both a scientific man and a literary one."

An Irish Medical Officer of Health with characteristic optimism used the book to try and get a £35,000 piped water supply for his district, as typhoid was endemic there due to infected wells.

Seventeen years later in an address to the Cambridge University

Medical Society,* Greenwood confirmed his assessment of Will's major work:

"If I had to choose the best contribution to statistical epidemiology made in England during the last ten years I should pass over the officials and professors and cite *Epidemiology in Country Practice* by Dr. W. N. Pickles, a country doctor. It is a very long time since research on that level has been done by town doctors. This is a model for research in social medicine".

The reviews of *Epidemiology in Country Practice* had scarcely appeared when the 1939–45 war broke out. The book can have made little impact in those few months, and indeed when the whole of the remaining stock at the publishers was destroyed in an air raid in April 1941 it looked as though its message might have been lost for ever.

War, when it came in September, 1939, was not unexpected; unlike that sunny August twenty-five years earlier. The war that now started had been feared and expected by millions since Hitler came to power in 1933. Indeed, in 1938 when Germany seized part of Czechoslovakia and civil defence workers were hastily mobilised to dig trenches in the parks, it had seemed to many that it had already started.

This time there was no mysterious telegraphic summons to Will. Once again the weather was hot and sunny, but they knew in Wensleydale that war had indeed come again when there drew up at Askrigg station a train full of children evacuated from Middlesborough and Gateshead, each child carrying a small suitcase and with a gas mask in a square cardboard box hanging round his neck.

* Brit. med. J., 26th January 1946

10

THE SECOND WORLD WAR

ALL OVER ENGLAND, in the country towns and the villages, coaches and trains were unloading parties of evacuee children in the warmth of an Indian summer.

The children were billeted on private families in the dale and were received with great warm-heartedness. As is now well known, it proved difficult in some cases for the country people to maintain a kindly and tolerant attitude to children, many of whom had come from some of the worst slums in England and whose cleanliness and habits were sometimes far below ordinary standards. In the end, however, even these difficulties, and the sorry state of affairs they exposed, produced beneficial results because they aroused public opinion about the need for better provisions for neglected children.

Some of the children who were evacuated settled down and stayed on for the duration of the war. They came to look upon the good people who accepted them almost as their parents. One childless couple in Aysgarth who took in a little boy of seven were broken-hearted when he finally returned to his home in Gateshead at the end of the war. Will and Gerty took in two boys from Sunderland aged twelve and thirteen who stayed with them for nine months.

For the Aysgarth doctors the reception of evacuee children meant more work; medical inspections, the treatment of head infestations, accidents and outbreaks of diarrhoea. A case of appendicitis and the delivery of twins to an evacuated mother occurred on the first day. The evacuees re-introduced diphtheria into the dale, which led to a small outbreak.

One of the Hawes doctors was called up and Will and his partner were asked to help out in his practice. Will's brother Jack, who had retired from practice in 1937 at the early age of forty-nine, came back and helped once again in the Aysgarth practice by becoming Medical Officer to the tuberculosis sanatorium.

In the summer of 1940 Will received a telephone call early one morning from Dr. Andrew Davidson. He told Will that a children's T.B. sanatorium had been burned down in the night, and asked if there were a big house available in the dale where the children could be accommodated. Will immediately got in touch with Gerty's mother, then an old lady of eighty-five, to see whether they could have the old family mansion, Thornton Lodge at Thornton Rust, for the children. Mrs. Tunstill willingly agreed, and forty children with various types of tuberculosis arrived that night on two buses with all their bedding and belongings. Strangely enough, many years before when Will had been chatting with Harry Tunstill about the ultimate use of the house the latter had said, "Well, it will make a very good sanatorium some day."

The Lodge provided a beautiful site for the children, and was later bought by the North Riding County Council from the Tunstills. It was used first to house the tuberculous children and later for mentally retarded children.

On one occasion when the tuberculous children were there, Will took an American doctor with some pride to see this beautiful place. Most of the children had glandular or bone and joint tuberculosis, derived in a good few instances from drinking milk containing tubercle bacilli. Will suddenly felt ashamed when he realised that the American physician had never seen these diseases owing to the much greater care the American authorities had taken to prevent the sale of milk containing living tubercle bacilli. More than ten years were to elapse before we had achieved a similar degree of safety.

Apart from the evacuees and the inevitable rationing and blackout, life proceeded in the dales much as before. The farmers became even more important members of the community and were encouraged by subsidies and urged by the War Agricultural Committees to increase the size of their flocks and herds and the fertility of their land. The two doctors continued work as usual, with visiting lists inflated by the evacuees and by a number of retired people with means who came from the danger areas and settled down in the quiet security of the Palmer Flatt and other hotels in the neighbourhood. They could get no locums now for holiday periods, and contented themselves with a week's holiday each year while the other doctor held the fort.

In 1940 Will applied for the Milroy lectureship. The Milroy lecturer is appointed annually by the Royal College of Physicians of London in honour of James Milroy, and the two lectures are normally delivered in London. He was successful and chose as the title of his lectures "Epidemic Diseases in Village Life in Peace and War". The lectures were, however, never delivered because the Royal College of Physicians' lecture theatre was damaged by a bomb. He could have delivered them after the war and might also have submitted them to the Lancet, which usually publishes these lectures, but, characteristically, he felt that they were not good enough for The Lancet and instead sent them to the University of Leeds Medical Magazine in which they were published in 1942.[11]

Will started by referring to the impact of the war on infectious diseases in the dale:

"When I wrote the schedule for these lectures, I gave as their title 'Epidemic disease in English village life in peace and war', fully expecting that much would happen to give point to this title, and anticipating with some dread that the wartime incidence of infectious disease would be sufficient for a lecture in itself. How wrong this was, everyone now knows.

"In few respects has village life been altered by war conditions and in respect of epidemic disease there is little to tell. Village life had indeed been altered already in some ways. Householders, a few gladly and graciously, many with resignation and some with bitter resentment, had accepted small, town children as guests (hardly paying guests) into their houses, possibly to bring with them disease and even death to their own little sons and daughters.

"Here is all I have up to the present to tell of the effects of evacuation on the health of the community in which I myself live:

"On 15th September, 1939, exactly a fortnight after the date of the first reception of evacuees, a little boy, a native child, fell ill with diphtheria and his brother became a victim four days later. These children, being newcomers to the village and actually unknown to me, had not received protective inoculation. An unfortunate chance had brought an evacuee to this of all houses and this child I was told had been suffering from a sore throat for a week. He was one of those to whom country life made no appeal and I never saw him as he went back to his home on 16th September, the day after his first victim was attacked and three days before his second.

"Impetigo, nits, scabies, enuresis struck terror in the hearts of the foster parents, but most unfortunately in this instance a sore throat was regarded with indifference.

"One epidemic was most definitely introduced by an evacuee. Our district seems fated to suffer from jaundice epidemics. I here produce a chart showing as the first sufferer an evacuee girl, her train of victims being thirteen in all, including three evacuee boys."

Having dealt with the effects of evacuation on the village, he proceeded to describe the special opportunities open to the country doctor to add to our knowledge of epidemics and to outline his own technique of investigations.

The lecture continued with an account of his experience and unique observations on the common infectious diseases. In several instances he was able to show that the incubation period of some of these conditions could be shorter than the periods given in the textbooks. For example, whooping-cough 8–9 days instead of the usual figure of 13–15; German measles 14–17 rather than 17–18; mumps 15–18 days rather than 21–35. He also reported that he had proved that infectious hepatitis could be infective on the fifth and seventh day of the illness and that he had arbitrarily fixed the period of isolation in his cases at two weeks.

Will sent copies of the lectures to a few friends and received some revealing and appreciative letters.

From May Smith, of the Industrial Health Research Board: "I always enjoy your writings as, unlike so much medical literature, you never lose sight of the patient in the disease."

From a fellow G.P.: "It makes me wish I had contributed something to our beloved profession, too late now I fear. Perhaps it couldn't have been anyhow."

Another general practitioner, Dr. J. A. Simpson wrote: "From what I can read between the lines you seem to be reacting to all the wartime problems with your unfailing good humour and kindliness and even evacuation has not shaken your equanimity – nor your faith in the good outweighing the evil."

From Professor, later Sir, Harry Platt, Manchester University: "I have read your Milroy lectures with great interest and with much profit to myself. It more than ever confirms my thesis that you are the last of the country doctors who document their experiences and from the stores of their knowledge make contributions during their life time. Whatever shape practice may take in the future we must see to it that it gives the fullest opportunities for men to observe, meditate and put on record their experiences."

From Sir Edward Mellanby: "My wife thinks you must be a very great man but of course I know better (at this stage you are heard mumbling to yourself 'I wonder what the old devil means by that statement?'). In any case anybody who has the instinct to, and who does, add to knowledge, especially about health and disease, is a man after my own heart."

In November 1943 Will was called urgently to the Grammar School at Askrigg and found the pupils in a state of collapse. Although influenza does not often cause such sudden and complete prostration he diagnosed this disease, remembering such cases in the 1919 epidemic and how, when he was a child in the early 1890s, his father had had patients who fell down in the streets with influenza and had to be carried home. He wrote to Greenwood about the epidemic which appeared to be starting and Greenwood prophesied that there might be a weekly death rate in Great Britain of about 200 before Christmas. In the event the rate rose to five times this figure. Will asked the authorities to close the school, and in this instance school closure did seem to be effective. At any rate there was not a widespread epidemic in the dale.

During the war Will kept in touch with Greenwood, who encouraged him to continue his epidemiological work. In a moving letter dated 21st September 1940 Greenwood wrote:

"I answer your letter in type, partly to be more legible, partly because the tapping distracts my attention from the gunfire and drone of enemy planes, which fidget one. Looking back on my life I am deeply conscious of faults and errors particularly of sciolism, a *restless* curiosity which has made me acquainted with many things but not master of any one technique and a rather childish love of scoring petty points. Perhaps in mitigation of sentence I can plead some gift for friendship and willingness to take pains so that my life has been happy for I have loved my wife and my friends and my dog and had pleasure in books and sums. No scientific note I have done will live, but I have stimulated others who will do something. You yourself have done something important and what you have done will stimulate others and the torch will be handed on."

Greenwood almost certainly underestimated his contribution to medicine. He is likely to be regarded in the future as one of the initiators of the great expansion of the application of statistics to medicine which is now taking place.

Will was now becoming recognised as someone able to give sound and independent advice from the point of view of the general practitioner, and in 1940 he was invited to join the Medical Advisory Council of the Nuffield Provincial Hospitals Trust. With this appointment he began to assume a role he was to fill successfully for the next two decades. It seems that whenever an important government or independent committee dealing with medical matters at the national level required the impartial advice of a good general practitioner they turned to Will.

He served for many years on the Medical Advisory Council of the Nuffield Provincial Hospitals Trust and later, when the National Health Service was introduced, on the General Health Services Council and its Medical Advisory Committee and on the Registrar General's Advisory Committee. He also served on the Cohen Committee on General Practice, which was set up by the Ministry of and Health which met monthly in London. Dr. Stephen Taylor, a large and benign Socialist who later became Labour M.P. for Barnet in the 1945 election and a life Baron in 1959, was on this committee. He and Will got on well and in 1951, when he was looking for material for his book *Good General Practice*, he visited Aysgarth to study Will's methods.

At the meetings of the Medical Advisory Council of the Nuffield Provincial Hospitals Trust, Will came into contact with some of the most distinguished doctors of the time. Sir Farquhar Buzzard, then Regius Professor of Physic at Oxford, was the Chairman, an office which was later taken over by Sir Ernest Rock Carling, a professor of surgery and an authority on hospital policy and construction. John Ryle, Professor of Social Medicine at Oxford, Sir Edward Mellanby, Secretary of the Medical Research Council, Sir Harry Platt, Orthopaedic Surgeon, Dr. W. S. MacDonald of Leeds, Professor R. F. Picken of Cardiff, Sir Henry Cohen and Sir James Spence, Professor of Child Health at Newcastle, were other members of this Council.

A deep friendship developed between Will and Spence. Like Will, Spence was a man with a love of humanity. Of both it could have been written as of Leigh Hunt's Abou Ben Adhem:

> "I pray thee then
> Write me as one that loves his fellow men."

Spence devoted one lecture a year in his undergraduate course to Will's work and would read out passages from *Epidemiology in Country Practice*. In his teaching Spence continually emphasised the immense importance of the consultation side of ordinary hospital practice. For this reason he would never allow more than two students to be present when he was seeing the mother of a sick child for the first time. He believed that more than that number would prevent her from speaking frankly about her fears and about the social and domestic circumstances which formed part of the whole picture. He was the first to introduce arrangements for admitting the mother of young children to hospital so that she could feed and attend to her child, take him to the operating theatre and be at the bedside when he was recovering from the anaesthetic. Because of his appreciation of the importance of these and other environmental factors, Spence became a leader in the development of social medicine, which was gaining momentum towards the end of the war and was to advance rapidly in the post-war years. Several others on the

Council were concerned with the advance of social medicine and the Nuffield Foundation, largely on the advice of this Council, played an important part in the development of these aspects of medicine by founding fellowships in social and industrial medicine and child health and in providing funds for the creation of professorial chairs in these subjects.

Will often drove Spence back as far as Doncaster after the Council meetings and they came to know each other very well. Occasionally Will would ask Spence to come to the dale to see a sick child and Spence often referred to these consultations as an education for himself.

Will also established a firm friendship with another member of the Council, John Ryle. Ryle was the first Professor of Social Medicine in the United Kingdom and had been appointed to a Nuffield chair at Oxford in 1942. Will had read his book *The Natural History of Disease* and corresponded with him about it, and Ryle recognised that here was a country doctor, who was able to take a naturalist's interest in illness and to make and record accurate and novel observations about disease and its spread in addition to carrying out his work as a doctor. He called Will "the Gilbert White of general practice".

Before accepting the Oxford chair of social medicine Ryle had been one of the most respected of the London consultant physicians. Some of his most frequent patients were doctors or their relatives. This indicates perhaps the highest reputation a doctor can earn, though not the most lucrative. In spite of the remark of a mathematical geneticist who referred to him as a "kid glove physician", Ryle was scientific as well as being a humanist. It came, however, as a surprise, at least to the London consultant world, when he accepted the chair at Oxford. He had unhappily only eight years there before he succumbed to coronary thrombosis after repeated attacks of angina pectoris which he bore with great courage.

During his few years in Oxford Ryle laboured greatly and successfully to lay the foundations of the new social medicine. He insistently called attention to the great difference in the health of people working in different occupations or social groups, he introduced mechanical methods of sorting and analysing large amounts of medical information from hospital records and surveys, and so made large-scale community medical–social surveys easier to undertake. He introduced new methods and material into the teaching of social medicine and he initiated an imaginative students' health scheme. The Nuffield Foundation arranged meetings of experts in these subjects in Oxford in which Ryle played a prominent part. Will attended one of these on the teaching of social medicine.

It was on this occasion that he asked Dr. Alan McFarlane, "What is social medicine?" and the reply was, "My dear Pickles, you have been practising it all your life."

The work of Spence and Ryle has been described because they represented the contemporary movement of social medicine and epidemiology of which Will had, almost unconsciously, now become a part. All three were humanists who were interested in and sincerely liked their fellow men, and all subjected themselves to the exacting disciplines of science. I believe that they were also agnostics who looked on death as the natural end not greatly to be feared. Will once said, "I'm not afraid of death. I'm annoyed, I never think of an after life."

One day he was discussing rheumatic fever with Spence and he happened to mention that although this disease was rare in his practice, he had one family in which it was unusually common and could be traced through five generations. Spence was interested and urged Will to publish an account of this family, but Will was reluctant to do this. Owing to one or two previous slights from editors, he had resolved not to submit any further articles for consideration, but only to write if invited to do so. However, Spence persuaded him to write an account of this rheumatic family and himself paved the way with the editor of the Lancet, at that time Dr. E. Morland. It appeared in August, 1943[13] and began in characteristic style:

"After many years in country practice, my experience of rheumatic fever and rheumatic heart disease had been so meagre that I felt justified in considering them locally very rare. It then dawned on me that the sufferers mostly belonged to one large family and more than once the disease was discovered before the relationship.

It was found possible to work out a family tree and to show that out of 53 descendants of a man – himself a victim – who died long before my time, 23 had suffered from rheumatic fever or had unmistakable signs of mitral stenosis. Besides the original victim I had to accept hearsay evidence of but three others, having myself attended and examined the remaining 20."

Although more recent work on the epidemiology of rheumatic fever and rheumatic heart disease establishes the dominant role of environmental causes in this disease, Pickles' account, and the work of other authors too, indicates that a tendency to rheumatic fever can be inherited.

In 1953 Spence developed a persistent cough and began to lose weight. After full investigation it became only too clear that he had developed cancer of the lung. When he knew for certain he wrote to Will in terms of stoical courage: "I go about my affairs. I feel inexplicably calm and tranquil about my fate. I cannot describe it except to say that it is tinged with the sense of relief which certainty brings." He died in May, 1954.

Today when we look back on the mid-nineteenth century, the great age of sanitary reform, we salute men like Chadwick, Southwood-Smith, Farr, Snow and John Simon who did so much to abolish the filth, the fevers and the premature death of those hard times.

Such are the uncertainties of history and fame that we cannot tell who, from our own times, will be saluted by those who come after us, but I believe that Pickles, Ryle and Spence will be among their number.

In 1943, John Gordon, Professor of Epidemiology at Harvard, was serving with the American forces in Europe. He had read Will's book and had been greatly impressed by it. He mentioned this to a senior doctor at the Ministry of Health in London and said he "would like to contact this fellow Pickles". "Very well," said the Ministry doctor, "we will invite him to London to meet you."

"No sir," replied Gordon, "I want to go and see him in this goddam little country town where he does his epidemiology."

Gordon was an epidemiologist of great drive and ability. He came to Aysgarth and stayed with the Pickles at Town Ends and among other things told Will that the value of his work was seriously diminished by the fact that he had not noted the ages of the patients whose illnesses he had recorded. At the same time he invited Will to visit Harvard after the war to give the Cutter lecture. He spent only an evening at Aysgarth, but as Will said afterwards, "It was a momentous evening for me."

After Gordon's visit, Will set to work on his old records again and with great patience obtained the ages of all the patients at the times of the epidemics he had recorded, going back over the previous ten years. To do this he took out with him on his rounds lists of twenty or thirty names of the patients whose ages he required and gradually completed the records in this way.

In 1944 he received a letter from the Ministry of Health which began:

"Dear Sir,
    I am asked by the Royal Commission on Population to enquire whether you would be good enough to help in the present stage of the enquiry."

The letter went on to outline a special aspect of the enquiry dealing with the extent of birth control and the reasons for family limitation for which Will's help was sought.

Will went to London to give oral evidence to the Commission. He was never late for an appointment and on this occasion arrived at the committee room in the House of Lords well ahead of time and before anyone else. As he walked up and down looking out on to the river, he felt rather apprehensive and wondered what he could possibly contribute of value to this august commission. He need not have worried for when he was called, Lord Simon, the Lord Chancellor, who was the chairman, immediately put him at his ease. "Dr. Pickles", he said, "I know your beautiful dale and I've walked every inch of it from Leyburn to Hawes." The evidence continued as follows:

Lord Chancellor: You are dealing almost with a closed valley?
W.P.:   Yes.

L.C.:	From Hawes Junction up to Aysgarth and Leyburn, a wonderful place, the gap where Mary Queen of Scots escaped?
W.P.:	Yes.
L.C.:	May I ask for how many years or for what sort of time have you been making observations that have led you to these conclusions?
W.P.:	I have been in that practice for thirty-two years.
L.C.:	Going from one end of Wensleydale to the other probably.
W.P.:	Yes Sir.
L.C.:	The children were really the old age pension.
W.P.:	Yes.

In the course of his evidence Will said he didn't think intercourse took place before marriage to test fertility. He also said that instrumental abortion was almost unknown and the use of abortifacients rare. The plant pennyroyal was used occasionally, however, for this purpose.

Lord Simon was particularly interested in the pattern of family life in the farming community. Will described this to the commission and emphasised how, if possible, the farmer tried to run the farm with only the help of his sons and daughters, regarding it as almost a point of honour to manage without employing outside labour, except at haytime. At haytime it was impossible to get all the work done without extra help and he described how it was the custom to employ Irish labourers for a month, or for the duration of haytime, if this were less, for a lump sum and full board. Eventually the Lord Chancellor concluded Will's evidence by saying: "I think we have exhausted our questions. I hope we have not exhausted you".

Will also gave written evidence to the Royal Commission:

"There has always been a great deal of selfishness among parents, especially farmers. They liked to keep their sons working for them as cheap and reliable farm hands and their daughters as domestic workers and general helpers on the farm and both were discouraged from setting up housekeeping on their own account.

"Much as I like and admire the people of the district I have been

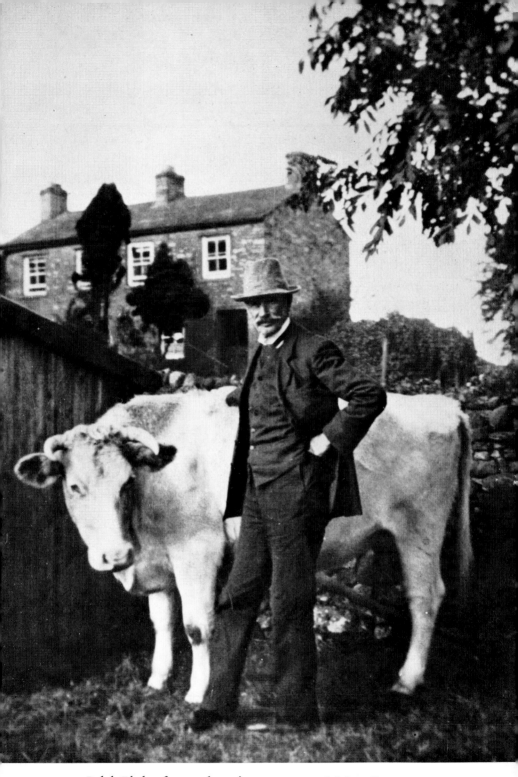

Ralph Blades, farmer, doctor's accountant and debt collector

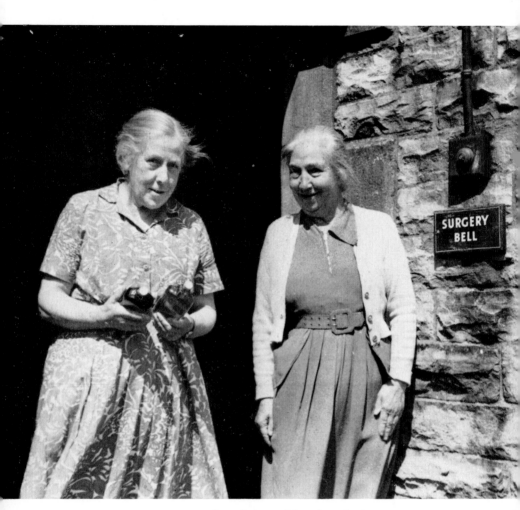

Madge Blades and her sister Jessie

disgusted with the spoilt love affairs and the disinclination to allow the young people to live their own lives. In the past the inevitable happened. The girl became pregnant and only on rare occasions did this not force the parents' hands, father and mother now bowing to circumstances and setting no obstacle in the way of him honouring his obligations. . . .

"There never has been much promiscuity, though every village has usually its loose girl or girls.

"Courting includes sexual intercourse between a couple who intend to get married.

"A rudimentary idea of birth control puts off the day of marriage till parents' convenience, i.e. ready to hand over a farm, or pregnancy supervenes. The local chemists say there is little demand for contraceptives."

Possibly one of the reasons why Will was asked to give evidence before the Royal Commission was because he had helped the Medical Research Council before the war in an enquiry into consanguinity in marriages. On that occasion Will undertook to inquire into the blood relationship, if any, between husband and wife in five hundred married couples in the practice. He found it a little embarrassing asking his married patients if they were related in any way. One farmer's wife replied with characteristic Yorkshire bluntness: "Do you think we're a bit funny then?"

In April 1944 he lectured to the Yorkshire branch of the Society of Medical Officers of Health and discussed among other things the chest condition well known to farmers which is caused by the inhalation of the dust from mouldy hay. The lecture was subsequently published in Public Health.[14] The disease, first described by a tuberculosis officer in Westmorland,* causes great breathlessness and disability and Will seems to have been the first to give it the name of "Farmer's Lung", as the following extract indicates:

"There can be few country doctors who are unaware of the ancient tradition of the countryside that mouldy hay has a baneful effect on the lungs of those who work among it. Most country beliefs

* J. M. Campbell, "Acute symptoms following work with hay", Brit. med. J. 1932, 2, 1143

I

are worthy of thought, and although I had heard this one for many years I was inclined to believe – what is no doubt true in some instances – that the condition was a temporary one due to the mechanical irritation of the dust. Looking back over the last 30 years, I can realise that if I had had that true humility and willingness to learn this, 'Farmer's Lung', as I think it should be called, would have been identified on not a few occasions and much suffering avoided."

He described one of the cases as follows:

"During January a message was received to visit another patient, a man thirty years of age, who lived at a farm at a high altitude where hay is got with difficulty in a rainy season. He was said to have had influenza but to have recovered sufficiently to leave his bed and attend partially to his work. I found him just returned from a short walk on his land. He was literally gasping for breath, he had a short hard cough and he could hardly speak. His face was congested and his lips were blue. At the time I thought I might find signs of a large pleural effusion but I was surprised how little abnormality I did find in his chest. The excursion of his lungs was small, just less than an inch. Breath sounds all over the chest were weak and there were a few squeaky rales at both bases. There was no dullness to be found anywhere. Had I on this occasion been at fault I should have been put right again, as both the man and his wife had decided on what was found to be the correct diagnosis."

He went on to say (and this was four years before the National Health Service was introduced):

". . . and as I am a great believer in Health Centres in country towns as centres for research I recommend this subject to a group of doctors working in one of them in the future."

On 1st January 1945 Ord gave Will six months' notice. He had bought a practice near Darlington. It had not been a happy partnership and Will felt a sense of relief at the prospect of its termination.
The war in Europe was drawing to a close and the end finally came on May 9th. The village took it calmly Ord, who had had a

night call, decided not to work that day. There was a service in the parish church and a tea-party at the Institute. Somehow the times were no longer suited to the wild junketing that had marked the relief of Mafeking or Armistice night, 1918, and the war against Japan was still to be won.

I I

POST-WAR YEARS AND A VISIT TO AMERICA

SOON AFTER THE end of the war, Sir Edward Mellanby, then Secretary of the Medical Research Council, and Lady May Mellanby, came to stay at the Palmer Flatt Hotel. He had become acquainted with Will at the meetings of the Nuffield Provincial Hospitals Trust Medical Advisory Council, and had come to Aysgarth for a rest and complete change. While there he put himself very much in Will's hands. A very well-known physician had made the diagnosis of "anginoid attacks". Either he had been unable to decide whether Mellanby was suffering from angina pectoris or not, or he was trying to fob off a highly intelligent doctor with a euphemism. Whatever his intention, the diagnosis had caused considerable anxiety.

Sir Edward and Lady May Mellanby became very friendly with the Pickles and Will would drive them round the practice with him, sometimes leaving them at a beauty spot from which they would make their way home on foot. Mellanby was thought by many to be taciturn and unapproachable, but Will's warm humanity seems to have penetrated the rather forbidding exterior of this remarkable man. Mellanby recovered to a considerable extent and returned to his onerous duties, which included his own research at the London Hospital in addition to the Secretaryship of the Medical Research Council. He survived another nine years following the "anginoid" diagnosis and made another important discovery in the field of nutrition by showing that the substance then used to bleach flour, agene, was the cause of hysteria in dogs. He was working in his research laboratory an hour before he died in 1955 at the age of seventy.

In July 1946, at the annual meeting of the B.M.A. at London, Will was awarded, jointly with Major Greenwood, the Stewart Prize of the British Medical Association. This was awarded him for "his researches in the field of epidemiology which provided a close determination of the range of the incubation period of epidemic catarrhal jaundice and the true light upon epidemic myalgia, Bornholm disease, and was a model for research workers in general practice."

After the meeting he met Sir McFarlane Burnet, the Australian virologist. Burnet was interested in Will's idea that the population in an isolated district like Wensleydale might, after a sharp attack of influenza, show a definite period of immunity for a number of years. Will invited him to Aysgarth for a few days and provided him with as much information on influenza in the dale as he could. Burnet subsequently published a paper, with a colleague and Will as joint authors, making use of this data.[18]

One morning while Burnet was staying with the Pickles, Will got a call to go up to Walden. In his own words:

"A farmer's wife suspected her maid was in the family way, but this was stoutly denied. In the evening whilst the family was in the hay-field this poor girl was seized in labour. If she could but walk two miles she could catch the bus to her mother's home and this she attempted to do. However, she got only a short distance and the pains overcame her. Climbing over a wall, she disappeared into a small wood and there her child was born. It happened to be a fine night and she wrapped it up in her head shawl and pressed it to her and kept it alive. A 'hue and cry' was initiated, but it was not until the following afternoon that she was discovered and she then picked up her baby, walked a hundred yards, got over a five foot wall and entered the waiting car, with the afterbirth, as I discovered, still undelivered. Never did a young mother make a better recovery".

Burnet was much moved by this drama of country life.

He and his wife Linda stayed with the Pickles again at Town Ends in 1950 and they became great friends. During this visit Burnet expressed to Will the view that he had done about all that could be done for epidemiology by the "notebook and shoe leather" method and that further advances in our knowledge of the spread of infection could only be achieved by the use of laboratory methods.

By this time Ord had left Aysgarth and Will was coping with the practice with the help of a new locum. He was a fat and hearty man who swore and cracked jokes and spoiled the cars belonging to the practice and often used them to go to the races at Redcar. He objected to working on Sundays, but not on account of any strong religious convictions. Will put up with him for a long time but finally asked him to go. Another doctor who had done a locum for Will suggested Dr. J. B. Coltman as a possible future partner. Dr. Coltman came on 1st December, 1946 for a three months trial locum. It was a hard winter and Will recorded one episode in these words:

"The year 1947 saw the worst winter for 100 years. On the day of the blizzard which ushered it in I rang up the home of one of my patients who was recovering from pneumonia hoping to escape the visit but to my dismay I heard he was much worse and his supply of penicillin which his daughter, a medical student, was administering had come to an end. I therefore set out on foot for the four miles there and back. The journey, partly on the railway lines, and visit took me more than four hours but my heart muscle, even at 62, must have been in reasonable trim as, after a whisky and soda, I was able to eat a hearty lunch. I had recently engaged a young assistant (Dr. J. B. Coltman) with a view to partnership who did a great deal of the rough work for me and I felt the experiences he had this winter would be enough to warn him off this practice. Far from it, he met all in a sporting spirit and decided to stay on."

At the end of three months Will was happy to take Dr. Coltman on as an assistant.

During this same winter there occurred a severe epidemic of glandular fever. The patients had a rash, much like German measles except that it was gone in a day. Will believed there was more than one form of the disease and reported this epidemic at a meeting of the Clinical Pathologists' Association in 1954. He described how he determined its incubation period as follows:

"There were two distinct epidemics. The second was introduced by a Royal Naval leading seaman on leave and like many of these people he was not in the least ill. I said, "I don't want to spoil your leave, Jack" – that happened to be his name – "but for God's sake keep out of people's houses". He took a broad view of this, or shall we say gave it a too literal interpretation, and I myself saw him escorting at least two of our prettiest girls through the village on, of course, separate occasions. He also was actually at a dance and three of those that attended it became victims at intervals of 18, 19 and 21 days, providing me with a nice incubation period".

Dr. Coltman married in June 1947 and it was agreed that his wife, Katherine, who was also a doctor would come as an assistant in the practice. This seemed to be a sensible arrangement. Will was now sixty-two and was involved in a lot of committee work and lecturing. It would obviously be a great help if the young couple could cope with the major part of the work of the practice and at the end of 1947 Will signed an agreement with the Coltmans under which they would receive the major share of the income of the practice. He made this agreement so that he could be free to attend the various committees he was on and accept any invitations to lecture that he might receive.

In May 1947 he accepted an invitation to address the Newcastle Branch of the Socialist Medical Association. Although Gerty on occasion regarded Will as a "rank socialist", he himself said he had no politics. From time to time he moved the vote of thanks to Sir Thomas Dugdale, for many years the Conservative member for Richmond, at the annual local Conservative Party meeting. In the field of medical politics, however, Will found himself rather more in sympathy with the aims of the Socialist Medical Association than with the British Medical Association. The former organisation since the early 1930s had been advocating a national health service, while the B.M.A. had opposed this idea.

Not the sort of man to enjoy controversy, Will experienced on his way to the Newcastle meeting feelings of despair. "Why did I let myself in for this? Why am I not lecturing on something I know something about?" he thought to himself. The majority of general practitioners had followed the lead of the B.M.A. in opposing up to the last minute the introduction of a National Health Service.

However the National Health Service Act was now on the statute book and it was to be implemented in the following year.

The meeting was held in the house of Dr. Douglas Gairdner. Thirty or forty other doctors were present, including Dr. Donald Court, who later became Professor of Child Health at Newcastle following the death of Sir James Spence.

Will had been in debt for many years after coming to Aysgarth on account of the money he had had to borrow to buy his share of the practice. He had come to detest the financial aspect of general practice which involved, in addition to borrowing money to buy a practice, the business of trying to collect bad debts, sometimes by employing debt collectors. For Will, as for many other doctors, a financial relationship between doctor and patient seemed to interfere with the doctor–patient relationship.

In his lecture to the Socialist Medical Association, Will said in talking of past conditions:

"The monetary aspect of the practice had to be of supreme importance and I can see that it might have become the ruling passion of one's life. There certainly was at the end of those twenty years a feeling of satisfaction in one's emancipation and I am bound to say a feeling of pride in at last owning the freehold of one's practice. But looking back I do not think that the heavy burden of debt was conducive to a detached attitude to one's work and the making of money simply had to be rather prominent.

"For many years, ever since the dawn of proposals for a National Health Service my colleagues, all country practitioners in virtually unopposed practices, have met in my house and in a most friendly and unofficial way discussed the various aspects of the subject. The attendances would average twelve and although rather more than half would fall in the upper age group the younger men were well represented. At the outset we felt that we were not now able to do all that we would wish for our patients in the way of specialists and hospital services and that, we were ashamed to have to acknowledge it, we could do a great deal more for those whose pockets were reasonably well lined than for those whose pockets were not. The hopelessly long wait that there is before one could

get a young man operated on for hernia or a child for the removal
of tonsils and adenoids would be instances.

"Many of us are tied to one hospital and when this is not a
specialist hospital one is at times in great difficulty through lack
of machinery of transfer. We felt that we were the people to
choose the appropriate specialist in reason, that is to extend the
privileges enjoyed by one's more affluent patients to all others.
We had hopes that a National Health Service would fulfill these
wants and we felt that the present time gave the profession a
glorious opportunity for putting its house in order. We were in
complete agreement that all our patients should have the opportunity of inclusion in the new scheme. We should personally
attempt to persuade all our patients to come in to it. We all
deplored the buying and selling of practices. About half of my
colleagues would be content to work in our present position on a
salaried basis and there was only half-hearted opposition from the remainder. We must all realize that there will have to be some super-
vision of our work and a periodic examination of our notetaking.

"At our latest medical meeting in Wensleydale we discussed the
form of health centre which would be of most benefit to our patients.

"I see before me the possibility of a service in which eventually
our patients will have their medical needs adequately attended to.
There is a long way to go and no one can state with assurance
whether our great country can shoulder all the financial burdens
this Government is arranging for it."

Douglas Gairdner tried to get Will to publish his contribution,
but Will refused as he did not want to get drawn into medical–
political controversy. Referring, years later, to the introduction of the
National Health Service he said: "I welcomed it with open arms."
In September 1947 he attended the International Congress of
Physicians in London and gave a short paper on "Infectious
Hepatitis". He was not often nervous, but this was the first time he
had addressed an international meeting and the audience contained
many world-famous men. He said to a friend afterwards, "It was
the sort of occasion when you stand up on the platform with your
knees shaking and wondering whether your flies are done up." He

need not have feared, his paper was well received. His power of transporting his audience to Wensleydale in the middle of a series of perhaps rather dull 'scientific' papers resulted in his contribution remaining in the minds of his hearers after many of the others had been forgotten. Lord Moran, who was chairman, said after Will had finished: "Dr. Pickles has again shown what can be done by general practitioners to advance the science of medicine," and the British Medical Journal of 4th October, 1947, reported: "At the International Conference of Physicians which was held in London last month, one of the longest rounds of acclamation greeted the contribution of a general practitioner, perhaps the only general practitioner to take any conspicuous part in the conference."

The number of visitors to Aysgarth was increasing, and that year included Percy Stocks, Chief Medical Officer in the Registrar General's Office in London, and Sir Wilson Jameson, then Chief Medical Officer at the Ministry of Health. Stocks was responsible for many remarkable epidemiological reports, including one on the geographical distribution of cancer of the lung and cancer of the stomach. In appearance a small frail man, Stocks continued to work on the epidemiology of lung cancer and bronchitis in relation to air pollution and cigarette smoking long after his retirement from official duties.

Will took Wilson Jameson on his rounds with him. Jameson was courteous and friendly with the patients, discussing farming with them very knowledgeably. He had insisted when he went to the Ministry of Health early in the war that diphtheria innoculation should be free. He had also insisted on direct access to the Minister of Health. In spite of his successes, including the near eradication of diphtheria, he became disillusioned with the Ministry as time went on and when he retired he wrote to Will: "It is twelve years since they tried to make a civil servant of me," and "I am a sad and disillusioned old man."

John Gordon kept his word about the Cutter Lecture at Harvard and in 1947 Will received an official invitation to deliver this lecture in April 1948. It was difficult to get dollars and visas to visit the U.S.A. at this time. Finally the Bank of England allowed Will two hundred pounds in dollars for the trip. When the American Consul

in Manchester asked Gerty in what capacity she was travelling she
replied: "As my husband's secretary". "Well last week I gave a visa
to a man's wife who said she was going as his mannequin," the
Consul replied, "I guess I can give you one as a secretary."

They sailed from Southampton on the Queen Mary on the last
day of March, 1948. In spite of a rough passage they enjoyed the
relaxation and social life of the voyage. On board they met Sir
Henry Dale, the President of the Royal Society, with whom they
became good friends. Sir Henry Dale introduced them to Dr. Gregg
of the Rockefeller Foundation and they soon got to know other
fellow travellers.

Dr. Mustard, the Commissioner of Health for New York, met
them on arrival at New York, and there was some merriment when
it was announced on the loud speaker that Dr. Mustard wished to
contact Dr. Pickles. Dr. Mustard took them to their hotel and they
soon found themselves looking down from their bedroom on the
nineteenth floor at the midget taxis and cars in the street below. They
were frightened to spend any dollars out of their allowance in New
York and on their first night felt they could not even afford a taxi to
go and see Broadway and Times Square. Later Will earned nearly
$1,000 from his lectures and got out of the habit of translating all
dollar prices into pounds, shillings and pence. While in New York
he addressed students at Cornell and Columbia Medical Schools.

From New York they proceeded to Boston to stay with the
Gordons at their pleasant home in Wellesley. John Gordon was
Professor and Head of the Department of Epidemiology in the
Harvard School of Public Health, and Will on arrival was asked to
talk to his famous class "Epidemiology 15" on rural epidemiology.
The following morning he joined in a "forum discussion" on
"Public Health in the Tropics". "To my horror," he records "I was
called to the rostrum and by the greatest good luck had a few words
and a Yorkshire story up my sleeve."

In the afternoon the Gordons drove the Pickles to Lexington and
Concord to observe the scene where the Americans had defeated the
British. This seems to be the regular first outing for British visitors
in Boston. They were also taken to see the homes of Emerson,
Hawthorne, Louisa Alcott and Longfellow. They spent an afternoon

with Dr. Theodore Ingalls, who for years had been keeping records of epidemics in St. Mark's school on rather similar lines to Will's.

Monday 12th April was the day of the Cutter lecture. Will had lunch, that is a hot dog and coffee, in Gordon's room at the School of Public Health and spent a quiet afternoon relaxing, as was his custom before delivering a lecture, in some room which was not in use. The lecture was in the Peter Bent Brigham Hospital and a large audience of staff, students and other "visiting firemen" had assembled to hear the sixty-three year old English country doctor. It is sometimes said that Boston is only half way across the Atlantic and English visitors seem always to be well received there in spite of their great number; many feel more at home in the capital of New England than anywhere else in the U.S.A. Will's voice had been considered weak in New York so they pinned a microphone on his chest. He started his lecture with these words:

"As I studied the long list of my illustrious predecessors who have presented the Cutter Lecture on Preventive Medicine I was truly grateful to the pious founder, that modest and yet forceful character, Dr. John Clarence Cutter, for the opportunity to visit this great country, to receive so many kindnesses from so many people and to find a truly New World opened to us on this side of the Atlantic. But what had I to offer in comparison with such eminent men? For I come to speak about very simple things, everyday happenings and elementary deductions drawn from them such as are within the scope of but a meagre intellectual equipment."

He then referred to his predecessors, William Budd and Peter Ludwig Panum and how they had also used the opportunities presented by sparsely scattered populations for the study of the epidemiology of infectious disease.

He described his first and only serious epidemic of typhoid fever in 1910 and the epidemic of infectious hepatitis in Wensleydale in 1929 which he had studied and reported so meticulously. He described the method of his work and the everyday happenings in the dale which promoted the spread of infections. He finished by referring to some old country beliefs about disease which have led to

important discoveries, such as the milkmaid who told Jenner she would
never get smallpox because she had had cowpox and the old women
who used to sell a concoction of foxgloves for treating dropsy.

The lecture went down perfectly. With his elegant and modest
style and vivid descriptions Will won the hearts of the medically
sophisticated audience and succeeded in transporting them in imagi-
nation to his beloved Wensleydale.

Knowing that he would be asked to lecture at centres other than
Harvard, Will had prepared three lectures to take with him to the
U.S.A. He showed them to Gordon who selected the one he thought
was the best and said: "Why don't you give this one everywhere?
It will be less trouble to you and no one will have heard it." Will
followed his advice.

The next day they travelled down to New Haven where they
were met by the Professor of Preventive Medicine at Yale, Dr. John
Paul, who took them to a cocktail party and to dinner. Will became
very friendly with John Paul and when he later visited London to
speak at the Royal Society of Medicine, Will travelled down from
Aysgarth especially to meet him again, and together with W. H.
Bradley and Ian Taylor, took him on a little public health pilgrimage
to see the home of John Snow, the nineteenth century epidemiologist
who showed that cholera was spread by the contamination of
drinking water with sewage.

From New Haven Will and Gerty went to Philadelphia, and then
on to Baltimore, where Will lectured to doctors in the Johns
Hopkins School of Public Health, surrounded by portraits of the
men who had made this medical school one of the greatest in the
world at the beginning of the century; Osler, Welch and Wade
Hampton Frost. It was the latter who revived an interest in William
Budd in the U.S.A., and caused his book on typhoid fever, long out
of print, to be reprinted.

From Baltimore they travelled to Washington and then flew to
Minneapolis. This was the first time Gerty had flown and she felt
beforehand as though she were going to have an operation. Will
was most impressed with the splendid student health centre in
Minneapolis University – one of the finest in the world – and they
enjoyed the parks and lakes of the "Hiawatha" country.

From Minneapolis they travelled to Chicago on the famous "400" train which travelled the 400 miles in as many minutes. Here they had an appointment with Commissioner of Health, Dr. Bunderson, the man who told Al Capone that he was bad for the health of the city. However the Commissioner did not turn up at the time appointed. "I can't do this ante-chamber stuff any longer," said Will, and he went off and spent a happy day with Gerty.

The next day they went on to Ann Arbor, a small university town with a population then of about 60,000 and a football stadium which could seat 90,000. Here they stayed at another fine university centre, the Michigan Union. Will lectured to the post-graduate doctors in the School of Public Health and they were entertained by Dr. Henry Vaughan, an authority on public health, and the Dean of the school at that time. The next stop was Battle Creek where Will thought he was to give a talk to general practitioners. However, nothing had been arranged and Will felt that the family doctor as we know him is a rarity in the U.S.A. Most doctors appeared to be trying to specialise in some aspect, such as cardiology or paediatrics. They left for Toronto a day earlier than had been planned. Here they were looked after by Dr. Neil Mackinnon and Will gave three lectures to the medical students.

Their last stop was Montreal which they had been invited to visit by an American doctor who had married a girl from Wensleydale. Unfortunately Will could not give the lecture he was billed to give owing to an acute attack of gastro-enteritis. This was the only lecture that he ever had to cancel.

At Montreal they embarked on the Empress of Canada for the journey home and they arrived at Liverpool on 29th May.

The two months tour in the U.S.A. and Canada, during which Will gave seventeen lectures, had been strenuous but immensely interesting and rewarding. They had met a large number of American and Canadian doctors and some of these had become great friends, such as the kind and wise Jo Garland, Editor of the New England Journal of Medicine, the Gordons at the Harvard School of Public Health and the Henry Vaughans from Ann Arbor. They had enjoyed the famous American hospitality to the full and Will had now become well known in medical circles in the United States.

12

THE NATIONAL HEALTH SERVICE

DURING WILL'S ABSENCE in the U.S.A. the Coltmans had faithfully maintained the records of infectious disease occurring in the
practice. Gerty now had to bring the charts up to date and to settle
down again to village life. To the Pickles, as to many others who
have returned from exhilarating trips to the U.S.A., it seemed as
though the brakes had been applied. The slower pace of English
country life was resumed.

Within a month, however, they were off to the Annual Meeting
of the British Medical Association, held in Cambridge that year.
The college in which Will and Gerty stayed for the Cambridge
meeting was not at all comfortable. "The single rooms were like
cells and the bathroom miles away," wrote Gerty, comparing them
in her mind perhaps with the American hotels in which they had
recently been staying.

There was much discussion about the National Health Service at
the meeting, as this was to be implemented within a week by the
Labour Government after years of discussion outside and inside
Parliament. Will gave a paper and hit the newspaper headlines with:
"Country doctor prescribes for the B.M.A." and "Down to earth
with Dr. Pickles". Both he and Dr. Horace Joules, who also gave a
paper, were among the minority of doctors who welcomed the
National Health Service and they advised the doctors at the meeting
to go into the new service wholeheartedly.

Will, in his paper, said:
"Many of us have had dreams about Health Centres and if they
are to become more than 'airy nothings' I can see in them a very
close link between the G.P. and the Public Health Service . . .

Child Welfare and schoolchildren examinations are really one
entity as one is the follow-on of the other . . .

"I am going to suggest that in some instances, especially in
remote country districts, these examinations should be conducted
by the family doctor . . .

"There is no reason why the district nurse should not work side
by side with the doctor in his surgery or health centre, doing
dressings and inoculations, and so economise the doctor's time.

"In one other way would Health Centres be of real value. There
are certain G.P.s who are well qualified to give health talks, and
those doctors working in a Health Centre who have the taste and
aptitude for this should be encouraged."

These remarks illustrate his remarkable capacity to detach himself
from the mêlée of medical affairs and to make accurate forecasts
about future developments. If the leaders of the B.M.A. at that time
had seen the new opportunities for better general practice which the
National Health Service offered as clearly as Will Pickles we might
not have had to wait for twenty years before they were firmly
grasped by the profession.

A year or so later when the National Health Service was in
operation he wrote:

"As far as one can see there has been no disturbance in country
districts of the doctor–patient relationship under the new régime.
This feeling is still there and will always remain there. No Health
Act, however imperfect, can destroy it". And,

"Dunbar and I always liked the National Health Insurance and
considered it a grave injustice that the benefits were not extended
to the dependants. We considered that Ministers of Health with
tongue in cheek did not proceed with this, as they realised the
dependants would be looked after gratis if necessary by the family
doctor, which was actually the case. What a far smaller upheaval
5th July 1948 would have caused if the country had shouldered its
manifest responsibilities thirty-five years previously. It was bad
enough in our area but the situation was quite impossible in some
of the depressed industrial areas, where the only source of remuneration was the insurance cheque. In one of our villages all were farm

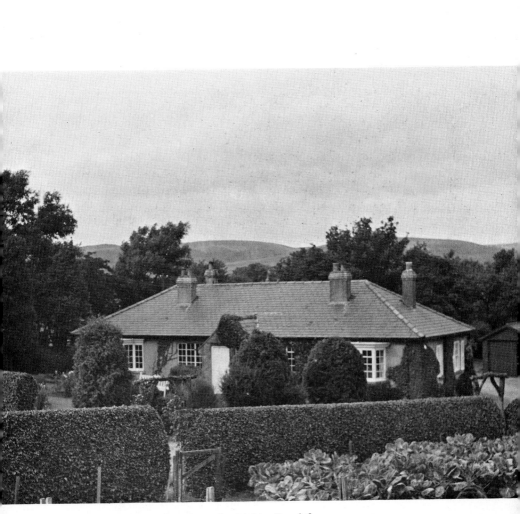

Town Ends, where the Pickles lived from 1922–1952

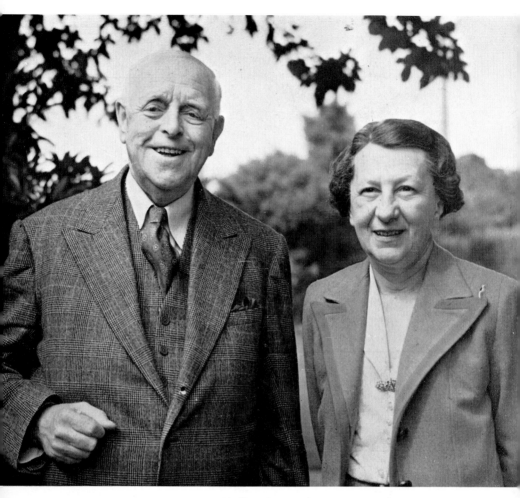

Will and Gerty 1951

labourers, estate workers or quarrymen, until recently quite inadequately paid. I was touched beyond measure when my book-keeper told me shortly after the inception of the 1948 Health Act that not one penny was owing from this village. They were not ungrateful, but in the past it was a sheer impossibility to meet even the small requests we made on them and we quite realised it. How delighted I was to get rid of the ledgers and daybooks and to grasp that money-making no longer entered into our work. What we didn't realise was how engrained in the public is the love of bottles of medicine and what a large amount of money is daily wasted because of this habit. Now, when all medical treatment is free, we are literally pestered to dispense and in an isolated district with no chemist, we ourselves are the victims as we have to dispense medicaments which we consider quite unnecessary, if not harmful. We must not underrate the psychological effect of these bottles of medicine. After all, they are reasonably cheap and complete X-ray examinations and extensive physiotherapy are very expensive, and to these we are also largely indebted for their psychological effect. The fairest arrangement is a full-time salaried service. I say this after years of thought and not always with this decision. I used to think it would encourage the slacker, but I have come to the conclusion that the real slacker is the man who takes 4,000 on his list and does the minimum for them".

At the civic reception given by the Cambridge Corporation for the B.M.A. Will was resplendent in his red and purple London M.D. gown and black velvet tudor hat. They met many old friends and acquaintances including Sir Henry and Lady Dale, Professor Parry, Dr. (later Sir) Theodore Fox, the Editor of the Lancet and Dr. Hugh Clegg, the Editor of the British Medical Journal, Sir Arthur MacNalty, Dr. Talbot Rogers (described by Will as "A very good man but doesn't understand country practice") and Dr. Charles Hill ("Damned amusing but . . ."). This was the first annual B.M.A. meeting which they had attended. They went to and enjoyed everything from sherry in the Mayor's parlour to the Medical Ball. On the last day they met the historian Professor G. M. Trevelyan, described by Gerty as "rather a faded old gentleman", who told

them he would write no more books. Following the Cambridge
meeting they went to eight of the next nine annual B.M.A. meetings:
Harrogate, Liverpool, Dublin, Cardiff, Glasgow, Toronto, Brighton
and Newcastle. On each occasion they delighted in the reunions with
old friends and made many new ones.

Although Will welcomed the introduction of the National Health
Service, he was quite prepared to criticise it and if need be take up
the cudgels for better conditions for the country doctor. He wrote
to Sir Wilson Jameson, Chief Medical Officer to the Ministry of
Health, urging a higher rate of remuneration for the country doctor:

> "I am fortunately in a position and at an age when the remunera-
> tion matters little to myself but I am passionately devoted to the
> cause of country doctors and I must do all I can to see that the
> country doctor gets justice and that the country people get
> adequate doctoring."

It is not known how effective these representations were, but
subsequently the country doctors' remuneration was substantially
improved by an addition to their income based on the distance the
patients lived from the doctor's surgery.

In November 1948 he was the chief speaker at the British Medical
Students' Association annual conference in London. After the lecture
he was taken out to dinner by the student officers of the Association
and one of them said to him at dinner, "Do you realise, Sir, that
there were representatives from every medical school in England
there today? You will get invitations to lecture to every medical
school in the country now"; and he did. In the end there were only
three out of the twenty-seven medical schools in the British Isles at
which he had not lectured. His lectures were usually very well
attended. On one occasion, on walking to the lecture room at the
London Hospital, he asked the chairman what sort of audience he
might expect. "Oh the place will be packed," was the reply. "They
will want to know what a country doctor looks like." Will always
remembered this remark on future occasions when he had an
especially good audience.

He gave the lecture "Epidemiology in Country Practice" more
than two hundred times. He did not repeat it word for word on each

occasion, but decided as he went along which sections of the lecture to include, the section on infectious hepatitis for example, the section on Bornholm disease, and so on. Each section had its more or less fixed introductory phrases and these led on to the stories of the epidemics that he knew so well.

Later that month he travelled to Glasgow to deliver the Finlayson lecture at the Royal Faculty of Physicians and Surgeons of Glasgow. He chose as his title "The Country Doctor" and described some of the epidemics he had observed and recorded in Wensleydale. There was an interesting reference to goitre.

"I myself have seen much of endemic goitre in the past, but I cannot explain why it has practically disappeared. Fresh fish has always been a problem in these parts and possibly additions to our diet from the village shop, such as tinned sardines, pilchards, and herrings, despised in our fathers' time, have supplied the necessary factor to the modern generation."

One is reminded of Balzac's novel *The Country Doctor* and the descriptions of goitre and cretinism among his patients in the alpine villages before the introduction of iodised table salt helped to eradicate these conditions.

This is one of the few references to non-infectious disease in Will's writings. Perhaps if he had been working today he would have been making observations on the habits and circumstances of his patients with rheumatoid arthritis, coronary artery disease, high blood-pressure and the other non-infectious diseases which plague us.

During the war Will had been the local representative of general practitioners on the panel committee and had arranged occasional meetings in his home for his fellow practitioners where they discussed the issues raised by the publication of the Beveridge Report, in particular whether there should be a national health service and if so what form it should take. After the 1939–45 war the meetings developed into regular annual occasions which came to be known as "Will Pickles' doctors' parties". Will found that some of the doctors in the area had never even met each other, and that these annual "parties" provided a good opportunity for promoting friendship and understanding. After the National Health Service was introduced they took the form of an annual informal lecture. The first was given by another remarkable Yorkshire G.P., Dr. Cockroft of Middleham, who gave a fascinating talk called "Two hundred years of country practice" in which he described the history of his long-established family practice. It was a great success and stimulated a lot of discussion. When Cockroft died in 1949 Will wrote the obituary notice for the Lancet in which he referred to this lecture.

"As a neighbour and friend for over 35 years, I feel qualified to write this notice about him, and, as one privileged to listen to his lecture on "200 Years of Country Practice", to write something about this remarkable practice, only the first holder of which was of different extraction. Those of us who were present at this lecture sat enthralled while he described the sequence of these rugged individualists and while he gave extracts from his own poems; and he was a poet of no mean stature. He traced the sequence of only five principals, describing their dress, how they travelled the rough roads, and what remedies they employed (all culled from extant practice records), what they charged for their services, and the detailed accounts they rendered to their patients – the very instruments, still in his possession, which they used.

"One must not forget his great work as M.O.H., his striving to bring pure water and decent housing to those for whom he was responsible for 42 years, and his especial concern for the care of the aged.

"His sturdy figure, his abundant white hair, and his singularly charming smile and hearty laugh, will remain long in the memory of those who knew him. It is probable he realised he had not long to live. He once said to me: 'A stroke is a grand thing so long as it does its job properly.' He worked until an hour before the stroke which rendered him unconscious and brought his life to a close..."

In 1949 James Spence gave the talk and called it "The day of a paediatrician". Later speakers included Dr. Ingram, the Leeds dermatologist who later became professor of dermatology at Newcastle, and Professor Stuart-Harris of Sheffield.

The meetings were held in the sitting-room at Town Ends. Before the time of the lecture the room was crowded and noisy with friendly greetings from doctors who had perhaps not met since the previous year. G.P.s from the dale like Eddison of Bedale and Adamson of Leyburn were regular attenders, and usually a contingent from Newcastle would come along including James Spence, Donald Court and Fred Miller. The late Charlotte Naish, another well known Yorkshire G.P., was usually there. In addition to running an active general practice she had brought up three children of her own, adopted another two and also found time to write a book on breast feeding.

The names of the speakers and all those who attended were recorded by Gerty in her neat hand. She had started the record of their visits and visitors some years earlier in her shopping book, but was now keeping a separate and more detailed account of all these happenings. The notebooks are full of accurate observations and discerning comments. Of one errant professor's unfortunate wife she said: "She drowned her sorrows in dress".

In October they drove over the Yorkshire moors on their way to Cardiff where Will was to address the medical students.

"It is such grim country we expect to see the Brontës peering at us over the walls", wrote Gerty.

Will thought the Welsh students were the brightest he had ever addressed, and a letter from one of them to him indicates that they obviously appreciated him:

"My visit to your home on May 10th, 1947 is a very privileged and happy memory capped only by the brilliant success of your inaugural lecture to the Welsh National School of Medicine which I was very thrilled to attend . . ."

In November 1949, Will met Aneurin Bevan at the annual dinner of the Society of Medical Officers of Health in London. He was struck with the way the Labour Minister of Health gave him the impression that he was just the person he wanted to meet. They talked about the Health Service which had been introduced the previous year, and Will told Bevan that it was suiting the G.P. quite well. Rather to his surprise, Will found that he liked Bevan and they went on to talk about Cronin's novel *The Citadel*. Bevan told Will that he had

nearly brought a libel action against the author because it appeared
that the secretary of the Friendly Society in the book was supposed
to be Bevan.

In retrospect there is no doubt that Aneurin Bevan was a great
Minister of Health. The fact that the Health Service was introduced
so smoothly, or indeed at all, was in large measure due to his skill
at negotiation with the representatives of the medical profession, his
willingness to conciliate and even to compromise on some aspects.
Sir Wilson Jameson, who was Chief Medical Officer at the Ministry
of Health during these years of change, told Will later, "I've worked
for him all these years and he is a very decent fellow."

The year 1949 was an exceptionally full one for the Pickles. Gerty
recorded the names of twenty-nine visitors in her diary and she
added, "This was one of the happiest times I remember in the
Aysgarth practice."

An important event in 1949 was the re-issue by its publishers of
Epidemiology in Country Practice, the Lancet reviewer wrote:

> "This book, now reprinted in its original form, achieved imme-
> diate success on its first publication in 1939 and by 1941 when
> enemy action destroyed the entire stock and type, was regarded
> as certain to become a medical classic. This judgement needs no
> revision after the lapse of years."

In May, Sir Thomas Dugdale asked Will if he would let his name
go forward to the Lord Chancellor's office for consideration for
appointment as a Justice of the Peace. After thinking about it for
some days Will declined on account of his age, sixty-five, and
because of his other commitments. Perhaps he also felt, as a man
who rarely judged or condemned anyone, that the part would not
fit. A letter from his brother Harold, written eleven years earlier to
congratulate Will on the publication of *Epidemiology in Country
Practice* was strangely prophetic. He had written:

> "I had always two great ambitions when I started practice, one
> was to read for the M.R.C.P. and the other to become a J.P.: and
> although my chances for either are now nil you seem likely to
> obtain both before you finish practice."

Will had got his "membership" and could, if he had wanted, have become a J.P.

Towards the end of 1949 Ronald Tunbridge, Professor of Medicine at Leeds, had confided to Gerty that the authorities of the University of Leeds were considering conferring the Honorary Degree or Doctor of Science on Will. Gerty was supposed to find out whether this would be acceptable to Will without actually telling him of the proposal, a somewhat difficult task. She kept the secret however, and when Will received the news one morning and called out "They're going to give me an Honorary Degree, Gerty," she replied, "Yes I've known that for *ages.*"

Soon afterwards he received a letter from John Ryle who had recently retired because of increasingly severe attacks of angina pectoris:

"My dear Pickles,

Another letter straight from your good heart, for which I am very grateful. Yes, the decision was not a happy one but inevitable. I would have liked say three more years to put the experiment more firmly on its feet. I saw with real joy, in the Times, the announcement of your forthcoming Hon. D.Sc. That and your invitation lecture tour in the U.S.A. are just rewards – over and above the thoughts and gratitude of many colleagues and patients for your very special contributions to Medical Science and practice. The letter of congratulation has been on my mental list but I have been going through a poor patch with much angina. However, nitroglycerine is a good friend (the only praiseworthy high explosive!), and I am very happy between whiles.

I only wish I were a little less marooned from my old friends.

Yours ever,

John Ryle"

In the letters of congratulation a pleasant note was struck by the warm friendliness of fellow G.P.s who were obviously proud of him. "It is so thrilling to read such an account about friends," one wrote.

The conferment of the Hon. D.Sc. was held on 19th May and the other honorary graduands included Lord Louis Mountbatten, Sir

Raymond Evershed (Master of the Rolls), Lord David Cecil and
Lord Lindsay of Birker, Master of Balliol.

Gerty was present and recorded the scene:

"The procession comes in. It is a beautiful sight. The honorary
graduands reach their seats in the front row of the crowded hall
and at last the Registrar reads out Will's name." The Chief
Marshall led Will to the platform and his Presenter, Professor
Matthew Stewart, introduced him, concluding with the traditional words:

'My Lord Duke and Chancellor I present to you William
Norman Pickles for the degree of Doctor of Science, honoris
causa'. He then conducted him to the Chancellor, The Duke of
Devonshire, who, taking him by the hand, said: 'By virtue of the
authority vested in me I admit you to the degree of Doctor of
Science *honoris causa* of this University.'"

Thus the University of Leeds honoured the country doctor.

At the formal dinner for the Honorary Graduands, Will sat
next to an old friend, W. L. Andrews, editor of the Yorkshire
Post.

Some of his patients in the villages did not quite understand the
significance of an honorary degree. "Dr. Pickles has passed for a
specialist," was one proud patient's opinion, while another is
reputed to have said, "I think he ought to have passed all his examinations at his time of life."

In August they visited a fellow G.P., Dr. R. M. McGregor, at
Hawick. He was working on the statistics of his practice and had
visited the Pickles at Aysgarth a month or so earlier to study Will's
charts and methods. Another G.P. who was stimulated by Will's
work on the epidemiology of infectious disease was Dr. Hope-
Simpson of Cirencester. He and his wife came to Aysgarth and
worked with great industry for several days, studying and making
notes on the records. McGregor and Hope-Simpson subsequently
published several interesting papers on epidemiology in general
practice.

In September Will received a telephone call from the sub-Dean
of the Birmingham Medical School, inviting him to present the

prizes at the annual prize-giving and to give the annual address to the students. Recording the event later he wrote:

"I said I should be most pleased to do so, although I found I should also be expected to propose The Medical School at the Dinner later. I never mind short notice. One's first efforts are often the best and one is apt to spoil these with too much alteration.

"By the evening I had the speech ready and only minor alterations were necessary, but every spare moment was spent in almost memorising it.

"My experience of speaking is of very recent date.

"When I have been asked to speak in earlier years I always said I was a doctor – not a bloody windbag and so I neglected what might have stood me in good stead. I must say contact with students and young doctors is a great joy to me and I do believe I can reach them."

At the end of his address he gave the Birmingham students an essential element of his medical faith:

"I hope I have not been preaching, but I am going to finish up with something you may think of this nature. Never use the word 'case' and never think the word 'case'. All those who come to you for treatment are individuals and often very frightened individuals and must receive the respect and consideration which one man owes another".

These were strenuous years for Will and Gerty. In addition to his practice and delivering lectures up and down the country, Will was on the Harrogate and Ripon Hospital Management Committee, the Central Health Services Council Medical Advisory Committee in London, the Northallerton Local Medical Committee, the Leeds panel on Infectious Diseases, a Somerset House committee on Medical Nomenclature and Vital Statistics and the Medical Advisory Council of the Nuffield Provincial Hospitals Trust. He attended thirty-seven meetings in 1950.

There was a more or less constant stream of visitors to Town Ends. Doctors and medical students who had heard Will lecture wanted to see him and the place where his epidemiological observations were made. Writing about this Will said:

"It is a great joy to demonstrate our charts and to attempt to answer their questions on general practice. I look upon it as a great privilege to have a few hours with these keen young brains. They think they learn something from me, but I know I learn much from them. So many young doctors are aspirants for specialism but those I see are hoping to enter general practice and I try to show them what a happy and useful life this can be."

In this way he probably influenced a good many young doctors to take up country practice.

At the suggestion of Sir Hugh Cairns, an Australian who became a distinguished brain surgeon at Oxford, the Australian Post Graduate Medical Federation invited Will to undertake a lecture tour in Australia and on January 18th, 1951, they went on board the P. & O. liner *Strathaird* at Tilbury.

13

AUSTRALIA, NEW ZEALAND AND
SOUTH AFRICA

THE WEATHER REMAINED good throughout the voyage until they
were approaching Melbourne, when a gale blew up and delayed the
ship for thirty-six hours, causing them to miss a welcoming party
that had been arranged for them. They finally docked early in the
morning and in the four hours before their plane left for Tasmania,
where his first lecture had been arranged, Will had to give several
interviews to the press and radio. He found the attentions of the
press distasteful, but on the Australian tour he had to smother his
repugnance and submit, because wherever they went the press had
always been forewarned and was there in force.

His first lecture in Hobart would have been rather thinly attended
owing to the rival attraction of race week, had not the doctors' wives
decided to accompany their husbands in force. Will noted that the
true specialist was then unknown in Tasmania. All "specialists" were
also general practitioners who were recognised by their colleagues
as having special knowledge in one branch of medicine.

From Tasmania they flew back to Sydney where Will had two
days of freedom from lecturing.

They then flew up to Armidale in the North of New South
Wales, where Will lectured three times in a week-end course and
had to deliver the first of many after-dinner speeches of the tour. He
was at the same time trying to learn something of the nature of
general practice in Australia.

"This town Armidale interested me," he noted. "It was a town
of ten thousand inhabitants with a wide district served by ten
doctors. Every one of these was working independently, everyone
was doing surgery, everyone had an X-ray apparatus, and an

electrocardiograph. I do not minimise for one instant the excellence and the enterprise of these doctors. They were doing a job of work far and away better than 90% of our G.P.s in England, but I think their system was wrong.

"I was struck by the small amount of visiting undertaken even in remote country districts. A provisional diagnosis is made on the telephone and if the condition appears urgent the patient is brought in his own car or an ambulance is sent for him to convey him to the hospital where he is retained should the bill appear a true one. All midwifery is institutional. All this makes for a vast saving in medical manpower and has become much more the order of the day since the acute shortage of doctors in the late War.

"I found it hard to assess the standard of general practice surgery, but I felt it was wrong that all and every G.P. should feel competent to tackle any, and every operation. Take for instance manual dexterity, what a difference there is among men in this. I know that in the past doctors in remote districts were compelled to undertake operations which our G.P.s would not dream of, but I do not think that it is at all necessary at the present day. I found very definite views on the efficiency of G.P. surgery from the professional surgeons."

From Armidale they travelled north to Brisbane, where the heat was intense, and at the first of Will's four lectures most of the audience had soon taken their coats off, whereupon Will was invited by the Chairman to do the same.

The officials of the Post Graduate Medical Federation had Will's lectures recorded on tape and his slides copied. The tape and slides were then sent to remote parts of the continent, including Thursday Island in the far north, so that doctors who could not possibly get to the lectures were able to get some benefit from his tour.

From Brisbane they flew back to Sydney, enjoying the map-like view of the coast all the way as they flew south. Here they had dinner with Sir Edward Ford, director of the Institute of Tropical Medicine and Hygiene, who asked Will for one of his original charts and a portion of one of his lectures to place in a glass case as a permanent exhibit in the medical school. In the neighbouring glass case was a black hat which had belonged to James Spence and which had become the mascot of the Department of Child Health.

From Sydney they went by flying boat to Wellington, New Zealand, and then on to Dunedin where Dr. Aitken, then Vice-Chancellor of Dunedin University, took them under his wing. Here Will lectured to general practitioners and twice to medical students and he was delighted to find that most of the students intended to become G.P.s and that it was considered "a real man's job in New Zealand and was properly remunerated".

Following this visit they had a holiday for six days with some of Gerty's relations in Havelock North and Rotahiti in North Island. Her nephew, Piet van Asch, an aerial surveyor, took them for a flight in a small seven seater and Will was thrilled to take the controls for a short time.

Back in Sydney again he was anxious to meet an old doctor of ninety-two who was said to be a great character and who was still in practice. Ted Ford took them to his consulting rooms, but a message came out: "I'm afraid I can't come now. I have a rabbit in the trap and hope to extract two guineas from her." Later on they met him and he drove them round the town. "This is our Parliament House," he said. "It is a rotten building, but quite good enough for the rogues that prate there." He told Will that he could never make up his mind whether to become a surgeon or a physician. He solved the dilemma by getting on the staff of one hospital as a consultant surgeon and on another as a consultant physician.

The next engagement was a week-end course for general practitioners at a small town in the hinterland of New South Wales, about two hundred miles south-west of Sydney. Doctors drove long distances to attend these week-end courses, and there were usually one or two other lecturers to share the burden.

These attempts by general practitioners, especially those working in remote country districts, to keep up-to-date and to maintain high standards of practice, greatly impressed Will. It was the great sympathy he had with the difficulties of the country doctor in keeping up-to-date that caused him to enjoy the week-end courses in the "outback" of Australia so much.

Back in Melbourne they renewed their old friendship with the McFarlane Burnets and were entertained by them in their home and at the Melbourne Club, whose architecture and atmosphere were reminiscent of the Athenaeum. Another week-end course followed in which he lectured at the little town of Yalloum, a hundred miles to the south-east of Melbourne. Then they had a delightful interlude at the home of a doctor who had given up medicine to become a cattle rancher on the shores of Lake Wellington, apparently a much more profitable job. The house had all the luxuries of a first-class hotel. Will and Gerty had their own suite of rooms looking out across the lake and farm boys were sent off on horseback to round up some kangaroos so that they could observe them bounding about in their natural state.

After two or three more stops for lectures they finally reached Adelaide by plane on a lovely evening and watched the sun set as they drove into the city from the aerodrome. They were impressed by the beauty and planning of Adelaide with its mile-wide belt of park land separating the city from the residential area.

From Adelaide they made the long flight over South and West Australia to Perth, from where they sailed for home a few days later. On the voyage home they stopped off at Colombo, but the magic of Will's first visit nearly forty years earlier had gone. The road to Mount Lavinia was now a modern highway crammed with motor traffic and lined with tawdry little "emporia". A visit to Aden in a temperature of $115°F$ in the shade was not pleasant. A few days later they passed through the Straits of Messina, and as night was falling they caught a glimpse of the awe-inspiring volcanic island of Stromboli. And thus to Tilbury where, in the tedium of queues and customs, the long voyage ended. It had been an intensely interesting and happy tour. A new network of doctors on another continent had heard about "Epidemiology in Country Practice" from Dr. Pickles himself, and those who later came to England made a point of visiting him in Aysgarth.

Towards the end of 1952 Will received an invitation from the Vice-Chancellor of Cape Town University to undertake a lecture tour in South Africa. The lectures were to be arranged in conjunction with the local branches of the British Medical Association.

This tour was not a great success. Will lectured in Cape Town, Johannesburg, Pretoria and Bulawayo but the audiences were small and many of the local doctors did not seem to have been told about Will's visit.

They greatly enjoyed a two-day visit to the Kruger National Park where they had close up views of antelope, springboks, wildebeeste and a magnificent pair of lions with their cubs.

In Durban they visited a hospital for Africans, and Gerty was shocked by what she saw:

"There are 1300 beds. It is very overcrowded. Old people are dumped here, the relatives leaving no address. Insane people come in – patients lie on the floor. Twelve women lay on beds in the labour ward. They are so quiet and patient, only their great eyes move. Five babies were born this morning and the average is 30 a day which works out at 30 tons of babies per annum."

From Durban they travelled by motor-coach on the long journey to Cape Town. The first day they reached Kokstad:

"It is a frightening town," Gerty writes, "natives with sticks as big as themselves peer into the hotel after dark. Few people would care to walk about the streets. I place my handbag in the bed at night."

and the next day:

"We drive through a Native Reserve . . . We visit a Native hut belonging to a woman with three small boys clinging to her skirt . . . It is a round hut with a mud floor and completely empty except for a bed (without a mattress) a heap of blankets on the floor, one hen and a very large dog."

and on the route to East London:

"The roads run on a shelf of rock in the mountain side and below the unfenced road are terrible precipices. We are just able to pass over the narrow bridge with no sides to it."

At last they reached Cape Town after a coach ride of more than fifteen hundred miles from Johannesburg. "I have my hair

shampooed and set at Madame Pompadour – 9s. 6d." writes Gerty
and one can almost hear her sigh of relief.

After a few more excursions in Cape Town they embarked on the
Edinburgh Castle for the journey home and that night Gerty records
some of her final impressions :

> "The happiness of the black man who shouts and jumps for
> joy – the dust – the fear of danger behind you . . . the beautiful
> white houses and farms of Dutch architecture – the jacaranda trees
> and the white doves of Cape Town. The tiny waists of the
> African girls and the lovely farm butter."

On the morning of 7th May they steamed slowly up the English
Channel in thick fog with fog-horns blowing and at 4.00 a.m. on
the next day tied up at Southampton.

Gerty finished her account of their South African journey with
a list of the addresses of all the hotels they had stayed at, the methods
of travel and the mileage between the places visited, a list of all the
doctors they met and their jobs, and a list of the lectures Will had
given. In addition to her natural powers of observation she had
developed the discipline of a scientific recording angel, which no one
appreciated more than Will. His own footnote to the tour was
equally down to earth:

> "From a medical point of view this journey to South Africa was
> a failure owing to no arrangements being made there."

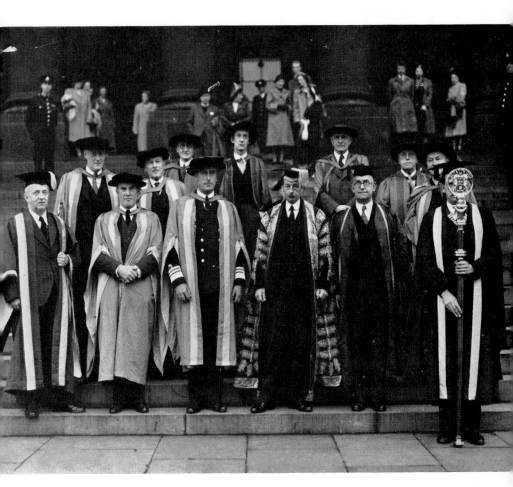

Presentation of honorary degrees, Leeds University 1950

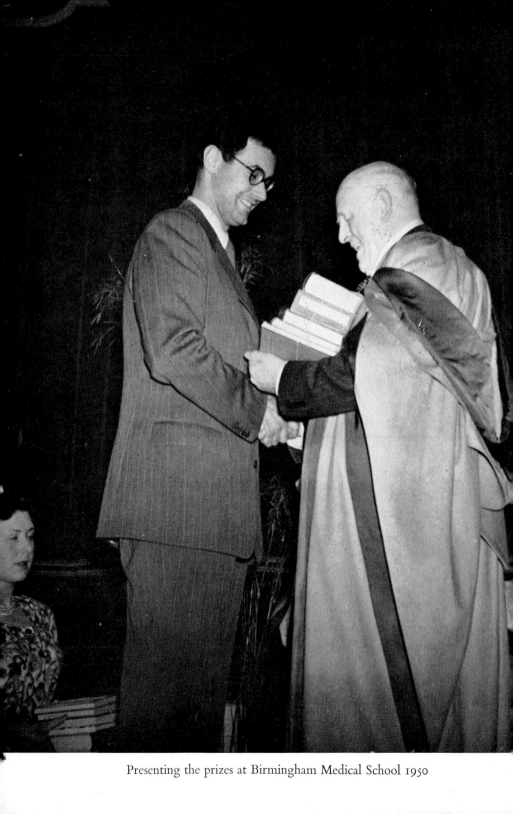

Presenting the prizes at Birmingham Medical School 1950

14

FIRST PRESIDENT OF THE COLLEGE OF GENERAL PRACTITIONERS

BY THE EARLY 1950s the National Health Service had already brought about great improvements in the hospital services by bringing consultants and specialist services into the smaller towns, but the conditions of general practice remained much the same. Nearly all general practitioners still practised from their own homes, often with poor examining and waiting-room facilities, and many had little equipment other than a stethoscope, an auriscope, a hypodermic syringe and a sphygmomanometer. Many G.P.s still practised on their own in isolation from their fellow practitioners. A highly critical report on British general practice by an Australian, Dr. J. S. Collings, describing some of these conditions had appeared in 1950.* He had written:

"The overall state of general practice is bad and still deteriorating. The deterioration will continue until such time as the province and function of the general practitioner is clearly defined, objective standards of practice are established and steps taken to see that these standards are attained and maintained."

A small group of general practitioners who were anxious to do something to raise the standards of general practice were meeting together at this time and discussing the possibility of founding a College of General Practitioners. The moving spirit among these was Dr. John Hunt. At about the same time two large health centres were being built under the National Health Service Act at Woodberry Down, Stoke Newington, London and at Sighthill in Edinburgh. These events were preparing the ground for change.

* J. S. Collings, Lancet 1950, I, 555

In Aysgarth some improvements were made. A room of the Coltmans' house was converted into a well-equipped surgery and the tiny annexe with its cramped consulting room complete with horsehair couch, and the little waiting-room-cum-dispensary which had served the practice since Will arrived in 1911, was now used solely as a waiting room and dispensary. Although the methods of practice remained substantially the same as they had been for more than a quarter of a century, Will no longer experienced that sense of isolation which had sometimes beset him before he started his epidemiological investigations which had brought him into contact with doctors from many parts of the world, and the stream of visitors continued.

One old friend who called with a special purpose was Dr. Stephen, now Lord Taylor, who was collecting material for a book on general practice. Some of his notes on the Aysgarth practice are reproduced here with his permission.

"I visited Dr. Pickles' practice in the course of a survey of good practices. His was the first practice I had seen where surgeries were of virtually no importance, almost the entire work being done by visiting. He or one of his partners normally turned up at the surgery three times a day, but often there was no one there. The main purpose of the visits to the surgery was to compare notes, to arrange for the distribution of medicines to patients seen on the rounds, and to collect messages asking for calls."

"It was Dr. Pickles' habit to make a round up dale one day, and down dale the next, leaving the alternate round to his junior partners."

"We went over the charts and discussed them at length. They were kept by Mrs. Pickles in a most meticulous way, by means of water-colour paints, in specially printed books; Dr. Pickles said he would like to see them going on for a hundred years. Mrs. Pickles transferred the notebook details to the charts once a week."

"The great value of Dr. Pickles' work lies in the fact that Wensleydale is a remarkably isolated community. It is therefore possible as a rule to follow the exact course of an epidemic. The most valuable single observation in any epidemic condition is the location of examples of 'the short and only possible exposure'. When one comes upon this, it is possible to work out the exact incubation period of any particular infectious disease."

"Besides the ordinary acute specific fevers, Dr. Pickles recorded every case of tonsillitis and other streptococcal infections, febrile catarrh, influenza, pityriasis rosea, herpes zoster and dysentery."

"Epidemic jaundice has an incubation period of about twenty-eight days, as revealed by a study of 'the short and only possible exposure'; its range is from twenty-six to thirty-five days. It is not uncommon for wives to infect husbands, but almost never do husbands infect wives. This Dr. Pickles attributed to the fact that a husband with early epidemic jaundice does not feel particularly amorous, whereas a wife with early epidemic jaundice may not feel particularly resistant."

"I tried to pick out the secrets of Dr. Pickles' success, and I reached the conclusion that he is a very wise man. He sticks to essentials and to simple principles. He observes exactly and carefully, without any speculative frills. He shows no tendency to jump to unwarranted conclusions. He has persevered in the work over the years. He has recorded his material meticulously, and has been much assisted here by his wife. His general practice has not been too heavy to fatigue him, so that his enquiring spirit has not been damped."*

During the next decade, with the increasing prosperity of the dale, most of the farmers were able to buy motor cars and as a result many more patients than before came to the surgery in the farmer's car or van or sometimes on the tractor.

Some people have assumed that Will must have had plenty of spare time in order to carry out his epidemiological investigations, and in a letter written in 1960 he commented on this as follows:

"I always feel slightly amused when my friends assume that I have had a leisurely life. This of course is true of the last few years (except for the delivery of more than 150 lectures), but really, previous to that, if my outside work has any merit it was at its best when I was working as hard as any G.P. ever does, scratching

* This description refers to the practice in 1951; much has changed since then.

an hour from here, an hour from there, out of my busy days and out of my allowance for sleep. When I wrote my first paper, on jaundice epidemics, this was particularly so. I have had sovereign health . . . I was always an early riser and non-stop worker, allowing about a quarter of an hour off for lunch. But whatever I say, I see a slow smile on the features of my friends – clearly they don't believe me."

Lord Taylor's book *Good General Practice*,★ which incorporated his observations on the Aysgarth practice, was published in 1954 and it undoubtedly stimulated some experiments and improvements. Its author himself played an important part in the creation of Harlow new town which included several health centres where a high standard of general practice has been achieved. In these centres the G.P.s' work was extended to include mother and child welfare clinics and occupational medicine in connection with the local new industries.

On 13th October, 1951 a letter which was to prove of great importance for the future of general practice had appeared in the Lancet. It was signed by Drs. F. M. Rose and J. H. Hunt and stated that preliminary discussions about the possible foundation of a College of General Practice were taking place in the General Practice Review Committee of the B.M.A. Many letters of support followed ,with a few against. The Lancet was cautious and advised against an independent body, suggesting instead that it would be better if the G.P.s' academic body be formally associated with the three existing Royal Colleges. The great majority of general practitioners who expressed a view, however, wanted their own independent college.

Dr. R. J. F. H. Pinsent expressed what many were feeling at that time in a letter to the Lancet:†

"General practitioners must achieve their college as their right and just due. They owe it to the memory of countless generations of predecessors in their practice that they accept no compromise title which carries with it the implication of inferiority to a college.

★ Stephen Taylor, *Good General Practice*, O.U.P., 1954
† R. J. F. H. Pinsent, "A College of General Practitioners", *Lancet* 1951, 2, 1185

General practitioners have been in a position of inferiority vis-à-vis the specialists for years, and it is this that they seek to amend. Were such an alternative title to be accepted, future general practitioners would bear the handicap of a decision made on the grounds of the political expediency of the moment, and they would have good cause to reproach those who lacked the courage to stand firm."

There was so much support for the idea of an independent College of General Practitioners that a steering committee was formed with the following membership: five general practitioners, Drs. G. O. Barber, J. H. Hunt, J. MacLeod, F. M. Rose, A. Talbot Rogers, together with Prof. J. M. Mackintosh (Professor of Public Health, University of London), Sir Heneage Ogilvie (Editor of the Practitioner), Mr. John Beattie, Sir Wilson Jameson and Professor Ian Aird (Professor of Surgery at the Post-Graduate Medical School of London). The Chairman was the Rt. Hon. Henry Willink (Master of Magdalene College, Cambridge).

This steering committee was subsequently replaced by a Foundation Council with slightly wider representation under the Chairmanship of Dr. G. F. Abercrombie. Sub-committees on undergraduate and post-graduate education, on regional organisation and research were set up and it was the avowed aim of the Council that the College should be the academic body for general practice and should take no part in medical politics.

The College of General Practitioners was founded on 19th November, 1952 with the stated aim "to encourage, foster and maintain the highest possible standard in general medical practice."

The first Annual Meeting was held in November 1953, when the chairman reported that more than 2,500 doctors had joined as Foundation Members. There had been no question in the minds of the Founders of the College when it came to selecting the first President. John Hunt proposed Will and the occasion was reported by the Lancet* as follows:

"It was common knowledge that Dr. Pickles had done a great deal for British Medicine. Many practitioners before him, including

* Lancet 1953, 2, 1087

William Budd and James Mackenzie, had retired from family doctoring when they became well known. But Dr. Pickles had resolutely refused to abandon his practice in spite of several temptations throughout the years. He would always be admired, not only for his original work, but also for the unshakeable stand he had made throughout his life for general practice and for general practitioners. . . .

"Dr. Pickles said he felt sure that the great general practitioners of the past would have approved of the foundation of this College. He was confident that there was no one present in the hall who did not look upon this as a historic occasion, probably one of the most momentous in the whole long history of general practice."

The Greek Ambassador then handed Will a gavel for the College made from the wood of an ancient plane tree from the Island of Cos, the home of Hippocrates. A year later the College had 3,000 members and twenty-two faculties in the British Isles. Membership of the College soon became recognised as a hallmark of the good general practitioner.

At the second Annual General Meeting in November 1954, Will delivered the first Sir James McKenzie lecture.

There were numerous distinguished medical men in the audience which crowded into the great hall of B.M.A. House, including Sir Harold Himsworth, Secretary of the Medical Research Council, Sir Henry Souttar, Sir John McNee, Sir Wilson Jameson and the Pickles' devoted friend Sir Ernest Rock Carling. "Will looks a lonely figure on the great platform," noted Gerty.

He started his lecture with a quotation from Jane Austen:

"You must employ the material which lies closest to your hand; you must contrive your story out of the simplest everyday matters as a small bird builds its nest from the mosses and twigs of the tree it lives in."

He went on to talk about his observations in Wensleydale on the modes of transmission of infectious diseases based on his records maintained over a period of twenty years of 8,808 cases of infectious illness.

At the end of the lecture Will was re-elected President of the College for 1954–55 and received a standing ovation which, as one medical journal reported, "must have warmed his heart".

From the platform Dr. John Hunt said:

"Little did Mackenzie think when he brought the infant Mrs. Pickles into the world that she would become the wife of a doctor who would rank with himself as the greatest practitioner of all time."

Afterwards a portrait of Will by Christopher Sanders, A.R.A. was presented to the College, where it now hangs.

The portrait was subscribed for entirely by general practitioners in the Yorkshire faculty of the College and presented by them to the College. It has power and distinction, but it fails to convey the warmth and friendliness of Will Pickles' character. His own comment on it was: "I don't look happy in it, and I always have been happy."

A month or two before the presentation the artist had brought the portrait up to Aysgarth for the finishing touches and after this it had remained on view in Will's house for a week. Each day twenty or thirty people came in from the village and surrounding countryside to see this austere painting of their much loved family doctor.

On the occasion of the second annual meeting of the College in 1954 a service was held in All Souls' church, Langham Place and Will was asked to read the lesson.

When he knew he was to do this he arranged with his usual thoroughness to read it beforehand to his clergyman son-in-law Gordon and to his Quaker friend Dr. Peggy Everett. They taught him to raise his voice at the end of a sentence. The lesson was taken from the Epistle of St. Paul to the Romans 8, 31–39:

"For I am persuaded, that neither death, nor life, nor angels, nor principalities, nor things present, nor things to come, nor powers, nor height, nor depth, nor any other creature, shall be able to separate us from the love of God which is in Christ Jesus our Lord."

At the end of the year he was invited to a B.M.A. Council dinner at which the Duke of Edinburgh was the chief guest. Will told him about the new College of General Practitioners, and the Duke with characteristic directness said, "I'm very interested in this College of yours, but tell me, why hasn't there been one before?"

In 1954 Will addressed the Association of Clinical Pathologists on "The General Practitioner and the Laboratory" and described the help that the G.P. epidemiologist and the laboratory epidemiologist could give to one another. He recalled how he had had to study the epidemiology of Bornholm disease and infectious hepatitis without the help of the laboratory. The part played by the Coxsakie virus in Bornholm disease was quite unsuspected when Will first described the disease in Britain, and the causal agent in infectious hepatitis has not yet been identified. Indeed in the early days he seemed to give more help to the laboratory workers than they to him. He described some of the curious requests he used to get from his laboratory friends:

"Dear old Marshall Findlay was one of the worst offenders. He often made the most extraordinary requests usually in a postscript to his letters. One of the strangest was this, shortly before he died: 'By the way' – and it is always 'by the way' with Findlay – 'can you let me have some rat blood?' I think it was in the study of choriomeningitis. I felt inclined to reply that I would catch him some rats, but he must come and deal with them himself as I had not the slightest intention of handling a fierce, difficult wild animal. But I thought better of it and tackled our Pest Officer who saw no difficulty in the proposition. He knocked the animals on the head, plunged a knife into their hearts and we were able to send Findlay eight specimens of rat blood which were sufficient for his purpose."

In the 1930s Will had used a private laboratory service for lack of anything else, but found this expensive and impersonal. He was therefore delighted when the Emergency Public Health Laboratory Service regional laboratories were established under G. M. (later Sir Graham) Wilson at the beginning of the war. He developed a warm friendship with Dr. William Goldie who was in charge of the laboratory at Northallerton and used these laboratory services increasingly and with great satisfaction. He ended his address to the Clinical Pathologists with the words: "Years ago I dreamed of the help we could get from a local laboratory and now the dream has come true."

In 1954 an article appeared by Will in the New England Journal of Medicine[33] entitled, "Sylvest's Disease (Bornholm Disease)" in which he suggested that the disease he had called Bornholm disease when he first described an epidemic in Wensleydale in 1933, should in future be known as Sylvest's disease because Sylvest "had done more than any man since the disease was first described to promote the knowledge of it." This was a generous effort on Will's part to give the credit to Sylvest. He also felt that the reputation of the Danish island of Bornholm might have been adversely affected by being associated with a disease.

It is difficult to get the name of a disease changed, and in spite of Will's efforts, this condition is still usually referred to as Bornholm disease.

In 1954 he received the Bisset Hawkins gold medal which is awarded by the Royal College of Physicians every three years to "some duly qualified medical practitioner, who is a British subject, and who has, during the preceding ten years, done such work in advancing Sanitary Science or in promoting Public Health, as, in the opinion of the College, deserves special recognition."

Will loved to relate how a few days later when he was showing the medal to a visitor from the village she remarked: "Aye it's luvly. Our Jack got one like that for darts".

At the "doctors' party" that year James Mackintosh, Professor of Public Health in the London School of Hygiene, talked on "Housing and Family Life". Mackintosh was a small, quiet but forceful Scot and possessed the fervour of the nineteenth-century sanitary reformers. He exerted a remarkable influence on public health education in the post-war years. He was less well known as a poet, but his book of poems *Airs, Waters and Places*, printed privately in 1961, gave pleasure to his friends. In his poetry, as in his lectures, he described the terrible overcrowding in the Scottish slums:

Life in one room
. . . but nothing done to find a house
They have applied for years and they are clean
Wholesome and thrifty; but too big
A problem for the authorities
Who think in terms of tidy sums
And averages.
Women of ease
Could you keep at bay
Bugs, lice and fleas
In a single room crowded, night and day?

Early in 1955 Will gave permission for *Epidemiology in Country Practice* to be translated into Yugoslav and later received the following letter from Dr. Branko Cvjetanovic of the School of Public Health at Zegreb:

"You are so generous in giving us such an excellent opportunity of publishing your book in Yugoslav . . . In our country we have still a number of infective diseases and epidemics and I think that many valuable data could be obtained if our physicians would follow the way you showed to us all. This is why your book will be of great value in this country, and let us hope, in other countries too."

15

SECOND VISIT TO NORTH AMERICA

IN 1955 THE B.M.A. held its Annual Meeting in Toronto jointly with the Canadian Medical Association, and this provided Will with an opportunity for a second trip to America. His old friend Henry Vaughan, Dean of the School of Public Health at Ann Arbor, promised to obtain some lecture engagements for him, and Harold Willard, a young doctor from Cornell who had visited Will at Aysgarth the year before in his quest for a more comprehensive approach to medicine, also said he could easily find audiences on the eastern seaboard who would be delighted to hear Will lecture. In June, when they were due to sail for Canada, a strike of ships' stewards occurred, so instead of the sea voyage to which they were looking forward, they had to go by air.

When the Canadian College of General Practitioners had been founded, Will, as President of the British College, had been asked to record on tape a message of congratulation which had been flown out for the founding ceremony. His voice at least was therefore known to many Canadian general practitioners and they were delighted to meet him in person and hear him address their College before the B.M.A. meeting began. At the B.M.A. meeting Will talked about "The General Practitioner and the Laboratory" on the lines of his address to the Clinical Pathologists the year before. As was his custom, the lecture was given without notes. Everyone was very friendly and one doctor said to Will after his lecture, "You're looking tired. Here's the key to my bedroom. Go up and have a rest." To another Will mentioned that he had become rather deaf. Thereupon the doctor went out and bought an ear syringe and syringed his ears for him.

To earn some of his expenses Will had promised to give a lecture

on "British Social and Medical Services for the Elderly" to a conference on "Ageing", organised by the American Gerontological
Society. He rarely strayed from his own field of infectious disease
epidemiology and before leaving England he had realised he knew
little about this subject. He had therefore consulted his friend Dr.
Lynn Sandford, Consultant Geriatric Physician in Sunderland before
leaving England. This must have been to good effect, because Will
remarked afterwards, "To my amazement I brought the house
down".

Dr. Vaughan, with whom they stayed in Ann Arbor, drove them
to Detroit where they met Dr. Tom Francis, the epidemiologist
who had played a key part in the successful trials of the Salk vaccine
against polio-myelitis. It was soon after this that the disaster occurred
when fifty-nine children developed paralytic polio-myelitis following vaccination. This tragedy, due to a faulty batch of vaccine, did
not detract from the great advance in the control of polio-myelitis
made by the use of vaccine, but it was a serious blow to the campaign at that time.

From Detroit they went by train to Hastings-on-Hudson where
they were met by Dr. Harold Willard. They stayed in the home of
some absent Scottish friends of the Willards, and had the opportunity
of "running" a delightful modern American house for three days.
Will also lectured to Dr. Willard's class of fourth year medical
students at Cornell.

In Boston they stayed with their old friend Jo Garland, who
published several articles by Will in the New England Journal of
Medicine. The Garlands gave an informal cocktail party, where
Will met John Gordon again. Gordon told Gerty that not only did
he advise his Master of Public Health post-graduate students to read
Will's book *Epidemiology in Country Practice*, but he also included it
in the list of "required reading" for their wives!

Later on that day they were entertained to dinner at the Harvard
club and after it Will lectured to an invited audience of doctors and
their wives. As he stood there in a light grey suit and bow tie, his
pink wrinkled face and bald head beaming on the audience, and
with a studied hesitation slowly unfolded his story of epidemics in
an English village which occasionally troubled, but never devastated,

the population, I watched the audience fall under the spell and tried to analyse the reasons why this lecture and its variations had proved so successful. Firstly, Will's appearance and modest friendly manner captivated his listeners, his voice and demeanour revealed so clearly the good country doctor. Secondly, the setting of Wensleydale, conveyed simply but effectively by two black and white lantern slides, the first showing the hills gleaming in the sun with white clouds blowing across the sky, and the second the same hills in winter under deep snow, helped the audience to project themselves into the scene. Lastly, the tales of the epidemics themselves were fascinating descriptions of scientific detection where the clue was usually some simple human event, a visit from a relative, an outing, or a drink in the pub.

Back in New York, Will and Gerty gave a farewell dinner party. The Willards came and Jack Weir of the Rockefeller Foundation with his wife, and the Waldies, in whose home they had stayed in Hastings. It was a happy evening and they were sorry to be saying good-bye to their American friends who had made their second visit to the U.S.A. so delightful. The next day they embarked on the *Medea* for home.

16

C.B.E.

THEY WERE MET off the boat at Liverpool by Patience and her husband, Gordon Clayton, who brought the news that Will had been elected an Honorary Fellow of the Royal College of Physicians of Edinburgh. Later that year he went up to Edinburgh to be admitted to the Fellowship and on the same occasion he was presented with the James Mackenzie medal for distinguished work in general practice. Will was the first to receive it and commented afterwards: "They didn't know who the hell to give it to, so they said, 'Pickles is an old fellow, let's give it to him'."

From Edinburgh they went to Liverpool where Will lectured to the Liverpool Medical Institution and Dr. R. J. Minnitt, the inventor of the self-administered anaesthetic machine for women in labour, presided.

In 1955 he also lectured to the medical students at Glasgow, Aberdeen and Birmingham, and gave B.M.A. lectures at Sunderland, Lancaster, Kendal and Doncaster.

Following his lectures he received many letters of appreciation of which the following from a fellow G.P. is typical:

"We all enjoyed you and your lecture so much, as it showed us what great opportunities there are for a man with keen clinical sense to advance the practice of medicine.

"I see very clearly how much more difficult it would have been, had you not had the luck – or the judgement – to choose a wife who was able and willing to keep those precious records, which if only imprinted on the tablets of memory would fade with the years. The G.P. is rarely articulate and many of his observations and tips on treatment are lost to the world and the youngsters tend to rely too much on mechanical diagnosis.

"You have shown our young men what can be done."

He went on attending and greatly enjoying the annual dinners of the various organisations to which he belonged, including the Society of Medical Officers of Health and the Leeds Medical Dinner for past students. He had attended the latter every year since 1934. For many years he also went to the local "Market Club" dinners in Leyburn which were held every other month. He would meet his Leyburn colleague, Dr. Adamson, at the dinners and thus kept in touch with what was happening in the lower end of the dale.

Like his medical uncles before him, Will was a Freemason and had at one time been Master of his Lodge. He enjoyed the meetings and dinners and regarded the masonic paraphernalia with tolerant good humour. He described the organisation as "para-christian".

In 1955 he celebrated his seventieth birthday. With his partial retirement from the practice and increasing disability due to arthritis of the knees, it seemed unlikely that he would be able to make further contributions to epidemiology. His arthritis, however, improved remarkably under a weight reducing regime to which he adhered strictly.

At this time he was in the habit of undressing soon after an early evening meal and then settling down in his dressing-gown to read or write for an hour or two. If a friend called in after dinner on a summer evening he would sit and reminisce over a glass of whisky, and when the visitor left he would come out to the front gate, or rather the opening over the cattle grid which served as a gate, to wave a cheery goodbye with his dressing-gown flapping in the wind revealing his brightly-striped pyjamas in the twilight.

In May 1956 when he was being driven by his old friend Victor Hamill, the proprietor of the local garage, to Northallerton to catch the London train to attend the centenary dinner of the Society of Medical Officers of Health at the Mansion House, he experienced a sudden vertigo. He said nothing about it to Hamill and managed to get his ticket and a newspaper, and to get into the carriage. On the journey as he tried to read, he noticed that words appeared to have their right-hand letters chopped off. He slept for most of the journey and on arrival he went straight to his hotel. He went to the dinner in spite of some persistent vertigo, which he hoped would not make him appear drunk before the evening started, and sat next to a senior Alderman who explained all the ceremonial customs to him.

He saw an ophthalmologist later about the attack and also his old friend Dr. Maxwell Telling at Leeds. The latter told him he should give up lecturing and "take life easy". He paid no attention to this advice, however, and gave many more lectures and went on several long journeys overseas. However, he regarded the "little stroke" as a warning signal and said to me some time after, "I think I shall not live long after that little stroke last year – but I'm not afraid." In fact he lived another thirteen years. A few weeks after the episode he and Gerty were on their way to the Annual B.M.A. meeting at Brighton. They spent a day or two in London on the way, where Will attended a dinner at Nuffield Lodge, a sherry party at the London School of Hygiene and cricket at Lords. "It is hot and sunny and the cricket is very slow," noted Gerty, "even the sparrows are asleep."

The B.M.A. meeting followed the usual course of ceremonies, social gatherings and scientific meetings. Gerty wrote less about it in her diary this year, perhaps through repetition the occasion had lost some of its charm, and it was the last one they attended together.

During the meeting Will went up to London to attend a luncheon given by the Royal Society of Health which the Minister of Health, Mr. Robin Turton, attended. He asked to be introduced to Will and they had some conversation. In comparing him with other Ministers of Health he had met, including Iain Macleod and Enoch Powell, Will said later:

> "No one was as nice as Aneurin Bevan. He gave you the feeling 'By Jove I'm glad I've met you at last'. All the others expressed the wish that you should meet them, but dismissed you when they wanted to."

Towards the end of 1956 he received an official letter intimating that he was to be given a C.B.E. He was delighted at this recognition of his work, but his pleasure at the honour was tinged with a

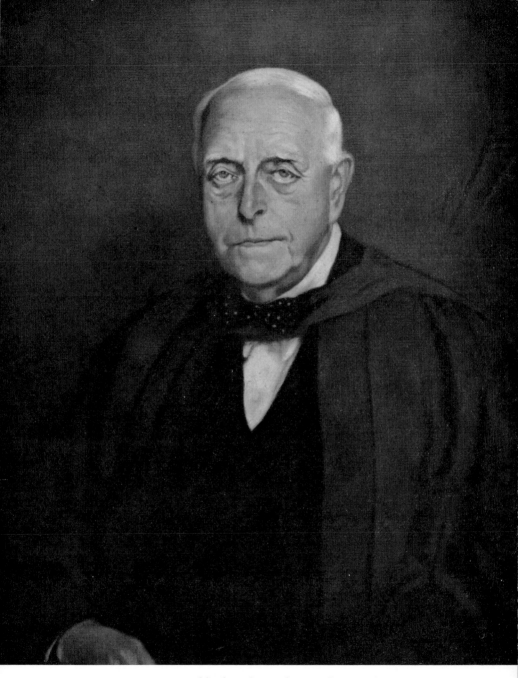

Dr. W. N. Pickles by Christopher Sanders A.R.A.

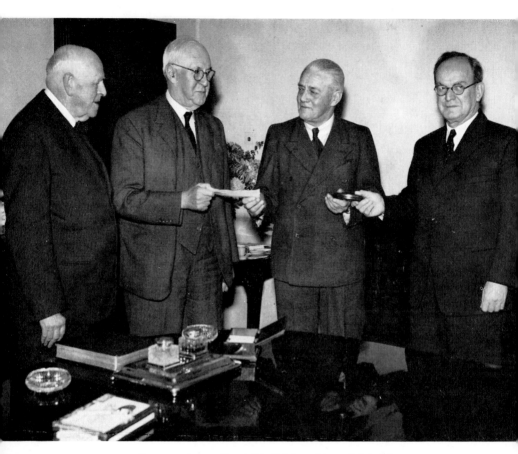

Presentation to Lord Nuffield on his 80th birthday

slight sense of disappointment that the opportunity of recognising the importance of general practice and encouraging general practitioners throughout the country by the conferment of a knighthood on the first President of the College of General Practitioners had been missed.

He had many letters of congratulation, including one from his American friend Dr. Harold Willard who wrote, "I can think of no one more fitted to Command the British Empire."

M

17

HOLLAND AND SOUTH AMERICA

IN 1954 DR. HAROLD WILLARD and I had started, with the help and encouragement of Professor Robert Cruickshank, then at St. Mary's Hospital, an International Corresponding Club for those engaged in teaching and research in social and preventive medicine. This later became the International Epidemiological Association. Will was a founder member of the Association and had contributed several articles to the Bulletin.

He was invited to give a paper at the first international meeting of the association which was held in Noordwijk on the Dutch coast during the first week of September 1957. The association was small but enthusiastic and fifty-eight members from Europe, the U.S.A., India and even Fiji, assembled at the little seaside town in a friendly and excited atmosphere for this first meeting. When Will and Gerty arrived at dinner time on the Sunday evening at the hotel which had been taken over by the club, doctors and their wives got up from their tables from all over the restaurant to greet them. Will's paper followed one by Dr. R. F. L. Logan on a statistical analysis of the work done by four Manchester G.P.s. With his natural modesty and his attractive and evocative use of words, he captured the attention of this critical audience of younger epidemiologists.

"If one sets to work to study epidemics one must have some simple technique and mine is extremely simple. I carry a pocket diary and at the bedside I enter under the date of commencement every sufferer from an infectious disease with the age and the village. My wife does the rest. Each one is entered on the charts which she maintains."

He was aware, however, that the chances of one general practitioner

making further important advances in epidemiological knowledge
were slight, as he continued:

"One man in one practice can do but little. I always feel that it is
the role of the country doctor to provide facts, which he undoubtedly can, from which others more skilled can draw conclusions, and yet some of the plums will come his way. I contend
that the mere 26 years in which I have been keeping records are
all too short and the information provided all too scanty. A large
number of doctors in general practice working in unison and
pooling information over a period of years could, and would,
produce many solutions which are badly needed. Since the
inauguration of a Research Group in our new British College of
General Practitioners, I really think we are on the verge of this."

Since Will said that, the College of General Practitioners' Research
Group has, in fact, published the results of several surveys carried
out by general practitioners working "in unison".

Jack Ustvedt, who was then Professor of Medicine in Oslo and
who was a great admirer of Will, greatly enjoyed Will's paper and
said to Gerty after it, "If we hadn't had a Dr. Pickles we should have
had to invent one."

Gerty kept a detailed record of the Noordwijk meeting:

"Sightseeing in Leiden . . . It is a lovely town with the canal down
the centre. The cafés are so gay everywhere. We have tea at a café.
A few people are playing cards and drinking wine. How cheerful
and different from England.

"We are driven by a medical student to Volendam, a fishing
village where everyone is dressed in traditional costume. The men
wear wide black trousers and sabots, the women long black skirts
and large coloured aprons. I loved it.

"We go on to see the monument on the Zuider Zee dam. Only
a road protects us from the North Sea on one side, and the Zuider
Zee on the other . . . Everywhere in Holland there is water. The
cows go across the dykes in boats."

There were also visits to Gouda to taste the cheese, to the flower
market at Aalsmeer, and to the Franz Hals Museum at Haarlem

where they saw the painting by Hals of the sour-faced women
governors of the almshouses, in which he was forced by poverty
to live.

The crowded week concluded with a farewell dinner and dance.
On the next day Gerty records:

"Many sad farewells are said. And so ends one of the happiest
weeks we have ever had."

and on returning to Aysgarth she recorded her final impression of
Holland:

"The windows clean; water, water everywhere; absence of
poverty; well-behaved children; the food rather dull."

In the same month, September 1957, the first annual scientific
meeting of the new Society for Social Medicine was held in Birmingham. Will was elected one of the first Honorary Members of the
Society, together with F. A. E. Crew, Wilson Jameson and James
Mackintosh. He was the only one of the Honorary Members
however who regularly attended the annual meetings, although he
never gave a paper.

In the 1950s, epidemiological research on the non-infectious
diseases and accidents became increasingly important and the
International Epidemiological Association and the Society for Social
Medicine in Britain closely reflected this development. Will's work
belonged to the era of infectious disease and these illnesses, although
still of the greatest importance in the developing parts of the world,
have become much less important, at least as causes of death, in the
Western world. The meetings of the two societies were occupied
more with papers on such subjects as heart disease, cancer, anaemia,
mental illness and accidents. Will was quite happy to take a back seat
and if the statistics were far more sophisticated than any he had ever
employed, no matter, his work was done and the record stood.

In December he took part in a presentation from the Medical
profession to Lord Nuffield on his eightieth birthday as a mark of
appreciation of his benefactions to medicine. All doctors had, at
Will's suggestion, been asked to contribute not more than five
shillings. There was a magnificent response, and Nuffield gave the

proceeds to the Royal Society of Medicine to found a Nuffield lectureship. After the presentation, Nuffield said to Will, "Now we'll have some food," and drove him off in his twenty-year-old Wolseley.

The second meeting of the Society for Social Medicine was held at Trinity College, Dublin, in September 1958, Professor W. J. G. Jessop was the host and the meeting enjoyed true Irish hospitality. Will shared a suite of rooms in the staff club at Trinity and was able to walk across the grounds and playing fields to the Moyne Institute where the meetings were held. Lord Moyne himself attended several of the meetings and functions and he and Will became good friends, later exchanging books. In the copy of *Epidemiology in Country Practice* which Will sent to Lord Moyne, he wrote one of his favourite quotations:

> "Pepys in his hour of peril to his brother-in-law Balty St. Michel collecting evidence in his defence: 'Pray learn from me this one lesson: to be most slow to believe what you most wish to be true.'"

Lord Moyne in the copy of his poems which he sent to Will wrote:

> "A much less useful book than yours, but I hope you may like to have it."

In 1959 Will, now seventy-four, flew to Cali, Colombia, for the second meeting of the International Epidemiological Association. The last stage of the journey from Bogota was impressive. The small two-engined plane could not fly over the highest snow covered peaks of the Andes rising to over 17,000 feet, but bumped about in the turbulent air between them. There was therefore a very close-up view of the great mountain barrier which prevented Bolivar from creating a United States of South America. Far below could be seen the river Magdalena on its serpentine and southward course and later, after traversing the central Andean massif, he could see the River Cauca on which the city of Cali was built.

On the way from the airport the hospital station wagon which had been sent to meet him passed through fields of cotton in flower and sugar cane plantations and he saw banana trees and bread fruit

and many tropical flowers. He stopped the station wagon where the
road passed over the Cauca river to look at the view. The air was
hot and still under the vertical sun. Down below the dark-skinned
women and girls were washing their clothes on stones by the water
and rinsing them in the river. Some of the girls were swimming in
the river fully clothed, their blue and red dresses fanning out in the
water and their black hair washed back from their foreheads as
smooth as seals. Across the river, punts loaded with bamboo trunks
and others with sand, were being poled towards the jetty to be
unloaded.

Will was entranced with his return to the tropics. He had not been
to South America since his service in the Navy in the First World
War when he had seen the sub-continent only as a series of brief
ports of call. Now he was able to see something of the interior. Cali,
a city of half a million, is 3,000 feet above sea level and, although
close to the equator, was not too hot. Will stayed with the other
participants at the Hotel Alferez Real. There was a grass-bordered
swimming pool on the roof and tables with umbrellas provided
shade for the members who assembled on the roof before lunch for
a swim and a talk.

Will was struck with the contrast between the luxury of the hotel
and the poverty in the streets around. Homeless and abandoned
children roamed the streets. Many of these had lost their parents in
the murderous raids of bandits in the surrounding countryside and
the children had gravitated to the city. It was a sad sight to see quite
small homeless boys take off their jackets at night, spread them on
the pavement and lie down to sleep.

The meetings were held in an air-conditioned lecture theatre in
the Faculty of Medicine of the Universidad del Valle and, as usual,
Will diligently attended most of them. He himself gave a short
paper. He stood up in an open-necked shirt and spoke without notes
although not without preparation. "Looking back on the years and
missed opportunities . . . ," he began, and gave a fascinating description of Farmer's Lung.

There were several interesting visits and excursions. On one
occasion a group of participants were taken round the hospital by
the highly intelligent and sensitive young Professor of Medicine. In

one corridor he stopped and opened a door with the words "We are not proud of this place". As the visitors entered the small ward they saw a dozen or so motionless children who had been admitted for diarrhoea and vomiting and nutritional diseases. The latter were mainly due to lack of protein and the victims were swollen up with oedema or showed the sores and discolouration of the skin and hair of kwashiorkor. Others were wasted so that their eyes appeared unnaturally large, their ribs stood out while their skin was shrivelled and could be picked up in folds. The hospital social worker told the party that one of her most difficult problems was to find homes for children who were brought into hospital off the streets by the police and for children whose parents just dumped them at the hospital and did not return.

Some of the excursions were too strenuous for Will, such as the afternoon spent trudging up and down the mud tracks in the shanty town of Siloe and the long dusty drive down to the steamy tropical rain forest, but he enjoyed the little dinner parties among friends and the hospitality given by the South American hosts at the luxurious country club, surrounded by patios, lawns and flower beds of gladioli. While Will sat sipping his drink in the great lounge some fifty yards long, looking out through the glass wall on to the swimming pool fringed with palm trees, professors from various medical schools in South America came to talk to the English family doctor and as usual Will showed a friendly interest in their lives and problems. One professor said rather ominously, "This place is going to be burned down," and on questioning he described the seething unrest in the country. He described how he had taught his medical students that certain diseases such as typhoid were due to drinking contaminated water supplies and that as a result some of the students had tried to persuade the authorities to introduce a piped water supply. The students were suspected of having Communist leanings and were expelled from the university and the unfortunate professor was doubtful whether he should continue to try and teach social medicine.

The wife of one of the Cali professors took Will shopping on the last morning, much to his delight. As he could not speak a word of Spanish nor she a word of English, the excursion was conducted in sign language. However, purchases were made and after passing through the usual tipping barrage of bell boys, porters and receptionists, Will and his old friend Robert Sutherland from Leeds set off together on the long flight home. This time they travelled via Caracas, the Azores and Lisbon.

A few weeks later, at the end of September, Will was off again, this time to Dundee for the third meeting of the Society for Social Medicine. After Cali, Dundee was cold and wintry in the east wind which whistled up the Tay.

18

HONOURED IN HIS OWN COUNTRY

IT WAS IN the University of St. Andrews that Will's professional forbear, Sir James Mackenzie, had, at the end of his career, established in 1919 an Institute of Clinical Research. Here, with the help of the neighbouring general practitioners, he had started to study the earliest signs of disease. Mackenzie believed that if only we could diagnose disease at its inception we could in many cases prevent its all too frequent and overwhelming advance. He knew also that the general practitioner was the only doctor who had the slightest chance of seeing illness at this early stage. Mackenzie's intentions did not, however, bear fruit at the time, partly because he died in 1925 but mainly because the conditions necessary for his plans to succeed did not then exist.

Looking back from nearly half a century later we can see more clearly what these conditions are. Firstly, it is unlikely that poor patients will go to the doctor about early symptoms which may appear trivial to them if they have to pay a doctor's fee. Secondly, there is not much point in discovering serious disease at an early stage if there is no effective treatment for it, as was the case with most serious disease in Mackenzie's time, and thirdly, special diagnostic techniques which were not then available are necessary for the earliest diagnosis of some important diseases.

With the introduction of the National Health Service in 1948 the financial obstacle was removed. Poverty need no longer cause the postponement of a visit to the doctor. The discovery or development of effective forms of control and treatment such as insulin for diabetes and streptomycin for tuberculosis, has made it very worthwhile to detect these diseases at the earliest possible stage and the introduction of special techniques for diagnosing diseases before the patient is aware of any symptoms, such as mass miniature radiography for pulmonary tuberculosis, or the cervical smear test for diagnosing early cancer of the cervix, have made Mackenzie's dream a reality.

In 1959 Will's old friend Eddison of Bedale died at the age of eighty-five. Eddison had joined Dr. Tom Horsfall at Bedale in 1902 and practised until a year before his death. Will, who had gone as an assistant to this practice in 1911, wrote an obituary for the British Medical Journal. In doing so he recollected his own early life in the dale and the difficulties the general practitioners of those days faced and overcome.

"A pair of broad shoulders, a tall powerfully-built frame, and a visage which breathed friendliness and good humor, a voice pleasantly modulated with well-chosen words and sentences, even in ordinary conversation – all combined to win the hearts of those who met this courteous member of our profession on his un-hurried path through life. Nothing ruffled him, nothing dismayed him, nothing daunted him. His life as a country doctor began when the country doctor could only with great difficulty obtain specialist help, when there were few aids to diagnosis, when surgical emergencies had to be dealt with on the kitchen table by the man on the spot.

"Francis Eddison always inspired confidence, not only in his patients but in those who were privileged to work with him, and by his exceptional hospital training he was quite capable of dealing with acute appendix, strangulated hernia, or perforation. All fractures were tackled as a matter of course. He used to say that one had to live with one's failures as well as with one's successes, and infinite care and considerable skill resulted in few of the former."

In March of the next year Will travelled to Northern Ireland to give a B.M.A. lecture to the North East Ulster Branch at Port-stewart. He accompanied a country doctor on his rounds the next day and visited with him a family of seven living in a typical old Irish thatched cottage. Will was delighted to find that the husband, a farm labourer, had in previous years worked in Wensleydale for several hay times.

On another occasion he visited Belfast to lecture to the Belfast Medical Students' Association. He was greatly amused at the tradition of the Queen's students that the minutes of the Association are read in an uproar of interruptions so that nothing can be heard, but when he started his lecture and warned them not to expect anything "erudite" they listened with rapt attention.

In May 1960 Will and Gerty gave the last "Doctors' party" in Aysgarth. These annual events, which had evolved from meetings called by Will and Eddison to discuss with their colleagues the proposals for the National Health Service at the end of the Second World War, had developed into annual social gatherings attended by doctors from up and down the dale and from still farther afield. James Spence referred to them as "a medical Glyndebourne" and the speakers included experts in epidemiology, public health, medicine, surgery and forensic medicine. The complete list was as follows:

1948   George Cockcroft of Middleham on the 200 years of his practice
1949   James Spence on "A Physician's Day"
1950   No meeting
1951   Stuart-Harris on "Influenza"
1952   John Ingram on "Common Skin Affections"
1953   No lecture – moving house
1954   James Mackintosh on "Housing and the Family Life"
1955   Philip Allison on "Heart Surgery"
1956   C. J. Polson, Leeds, on "Signs of Violence"
1957   W. H. Bradley, Ministry of Health, on "Recent Epidemics"
1958   Frazer Brockington on his "Eastern Journey"
1959   Sir John McNee on "Diseases of the Liver: a 40 years retrospect"
1960   *Final Lecture* – Henry Miller, Newcastle, on "Accident Neuroses"

At first the meetings were held in their old home, Town Ends, but later, after they had moved to the smaller bungalow, the lecture was given at the Institute in the village followed by tea at the

bungalow. The weather seems nearly always to have been fine and
so the guests could overflow into the little garden.

Soon after the last doctors' party, Dr. Adamson of Leyburn had
come to see Will and Gerty to tell them that their medical friends
wished to give them a dinner and presentation, and on 22nd October,
1960 there took place a memorable gathering in a hotel in Leyburn.
Of the seventy who had been invited, sixty-five assembled at the
hotel to show their appreciation for what Will and Gerty had done
for the profession in Wensleydale. It was a dinner-jacket occasion,
starting off with sherry and cocktails, and after dinner Dr. William
Goldie rose to make the presentation. Some of the things that were
said on that occasion were taken down by Dr. Peggy Everett.
Dr. Goldie said:

"To-night we try to express our gratitude to Will and Gertrude
Pickles who have so often been our hosts. Will is one who is
known wherever medicine is practised – as one of the great
doctors of his generation . . .

"Then he came to this loveliest of all dales . . . Many had not
been in a train, the car had not begun its destructive career, it was
the day of horseback . . .

"We, nowadays, need all our costly apparatus; Will arrived
with ears and eyes only; native wit, insatiable curiosity, almost
nosiness . . .

"He has shown that general practice need not be a dull routine.

"Honours have been showered on him, C.B.E., M.R.C.P.,
F.R.C.P.Ed., Milroy Lecturer, Cutter (Harvard) Lecturer, James
Mackenzie Medal, First President of the College of G.P.s (and
more that do not come instantly to my mind), but he still remains
the same modest, loveable W.P.

"We thank you and will remember those gatherings all our
lives.

"W.P. reminds us sometimes of Chaucer's Monk: 'His head
was bald and shone as any glass and eke his face as he had been
anoint.'

"But perhaps more of his Knight, and those words, 'He was a
verray parfit gentil knight.'"

In his reply Will said:

" 'There is no refreshment of the spirit equal to the companionship of friends.'

"So wrote James Spence after one of the parties which led up to this most delightful occasion. Everyone here knows what a pleasure it has been to us to welcome our friends year by year to our Doctors' Parties, and how sad we are that they must cease."

In the course of his speech Will referred to a previous Wensleydale dinner:

"In the nineties, one Dick Heseltine, Landlord of the George and Dragon Hotel, Aysgarth, a hostelry well known to you, arrived late and was still eating when 'God save the Queen' was played. He went on eating. 'Get up, Dick, don't you know it's "God save the Queen"?' Dick never moved and went on stolidly eating. When he had finished he turned to the Chairman and said, 'Mr. Winn, there isn't a loyaller man in Wensleydale, but I were thrang wit' duck'."

and Will continued:

"What a gathering it is. It is really a remarkable thing to see in this remote little market town so many varieties of doctors. I will attempt to enumerate them with, mind you, no attempt at precedence.

"There are physicians and surgeons including one, we are most pleased to see, from the other side of the Atlantic, and G.P.s.

"There are dermatologists, paediatricians and a geriatrician.

"There is a Principal Medical Officer from the Ministry of Health, a Superintendent of a Fever Hospital, a Lecturer in Social Medicine and a Specialist in anaesthetics.

"And you have done a delightful thing. You have persuaded your wives to accompany you to complete the picture, with their bright faces, their happy melodious laughter and their pretty frocks, bless them!

"Thank you all for this evening, I believe the happiest of our lives."

Dr. Adamson who had organised the dinner said:

"We are so busy now we have lost many of the gracious ways of life; then – the local doctors all called and left their cards. We must re-establish ourselves in the same friendly ways again if there is to be any hope for our working together successfully in the medical services."

Dr. Adamson finished his tribute with these words:

"It has been grand to have known you and to have shared this great regard for the importance of the doctor–doctor relationship expressed in these annual dales gatherings."

Several of the other guests at the dinner paid tribute to Will.

Dr. W. S. MacDonald said:

"I speak in a state of humility. I represent the periphery of a distinguished centre. I think of the people here tonight in spirit – Sir Farquhar Buzzard, Sir Ernest Rock Carling. No prophet has received greater honour in his own country than has Will Pickles tonight."

Dr. Robert Sutherland, referring to Will's role in the Society for Social Medicine and the International Epidemiological Association, said:

". . . at those meetings he sits quietly in his corner and the world comes to him for his always delightful company and to draw on his stores of wisdom. His contribution to epidemiology will be regarded as a classic in ages to come."

Dr. Ollerenshaw of Skipton, one of the founders of the College of General Practitioners, added his tribute:

"I find myself surprised and terrified on my feet. But I am pushed to my feet by some people not here. The College of General Practitioners would not forgive me if I did not say something in their name. I was one of the members of its Foundation Council and I know there was absolutely no argument as to who the first President should be.

"The people who belong to the inarticulate mass of G.P.s have made their voice heard this evening."

19

THE LAST YEARS

AT THE END of August 1961, Will left for Korcula, an island off the coast of Yugoslavia, for the third international meeting of the International Epidemiological Association. He took the night flight to Venice and found himself chugging along the Grand Canal in the *vaporetto* before dawn to his hotel. The city of swarming tourists was momentarily silent, and the palaces rose grey and indistinct beside the lapping water. After a few hours' sleep in his hotel near St. Mark's Square, he got up to see the Ducal Palace shining in the sun like a wedding cake and he was fascinated by the incessant movement of motor-boats, gondolas and steamers on the lagoon.

The twenty-four hour sea trip down the Adriatic Coast was delightful. The sun shone all the time, but there was a cool persistent wind which flecked with white the dark blue sea. They called at Split and Hvar before arriving at the beautiful old town on the island of Korcula.

The members of the Association fully occupied a new hotel which had not been begun when the first bookings were made. The atmosphere was intimate and friendly, and Will enjoyed it all, especially sitting on the terrace of the restaurant looking out across the sea to the other islands and talking to his many friends.

The scientific meetings were held in the small municipal hall and the municipality, which had never before had to cope with an international medical meeting, went to great pains to black out the hall so that slides could be shown. They also provided thick black Turkish coffee in the intervals, rowing boats for the children, a flotilla of motor launches for an outing to some other islands for the whole conference, and an open-air reception by moonlight in the town's ancient mediaeval courtyard.

The week passed quickly in these beautiful surroundings.

In November he attended the annual meeting of the College of General Practitioners and was presented with the Foundation Council Award, which consisted of a silver replica of the College gavel with an entwined snake on an ebony plinth. The citation said " for work of the highest merit in the realm of general practice and for service of the greatest distinction to the cause of general practice."

He was now seventy-six, but still active, although to a limited extent, in his practice.

The following March he took part in a ceremony to mark the 250th anniversary of the birth of his famous Wensleydale predecessor, the Quaker physician John Fothergill, who was born at Carr End overlooking Semerwater, on 10th March, 1712. John Fothergill, unlike Will, had left his native dale to make his name and a large fortune in London. He is remembered in medical history for his *Account of the Sore Throat*, and as the moving spirit in the foundation of one of the earliest medical societies of London, The Society of Physicians. He also described artificial respiration, popularised the use of coffee in Britain, and founded Ackworth School. Will described the scene for the New England Journal of Medicine thus:

"A drive on a wintry afternoon, complete with that cold thaw wind in which Wensleydale specializes, a breathtaking glimpse of lovely little Lake Semerwater, and a trudge uphill over the softening snow to a tiny Friends' meetinghouse were the preliminaries to a memorable gathering. Sixty lovers of the dale met on March 10, two days after the two hundred and fiftieth anniversary of his birth, to do honour to the memory of Dr. John Fothergill, amid dignified, sober surroundings, old-oak panelling and old-oak benches in a well-proportioned Georgian room, within a mile of his birthplace.

"Called upon by the Quaker clerk, who had himself read, 'Let us now praise famous men', from Ecclesiasticus, first a retired schoolmistress, wife of a descendant of John's brother, went a long way with her vivid descriptions of him and excerpts from his letters to bring him to life. Then a young physician from a London

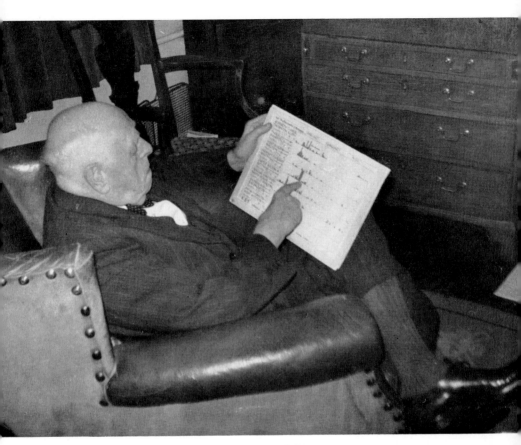

Will on his 80th birthday

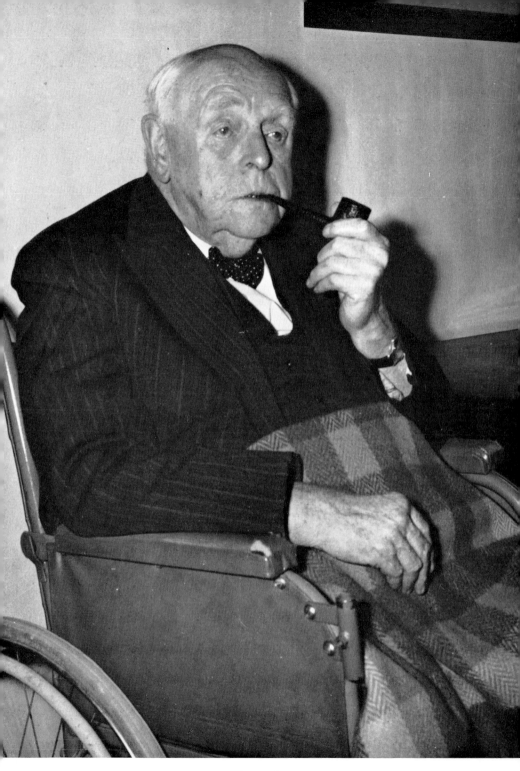

May 1967

hospital, who was brought up as a child in this district, described attractively and fluently his many medical achievements.

"Lastly, the old country doctor attempted to round off the proceedings with thanks and congratulations to the speakers, references to John's friends, Lettsom and William Hillary (this last born within two miles of the meeting) and by claiming John Fothergill as Wensleydale's greatest son."

The other Wensleydale physician mentioned by Will was William Hillary (1697–1763), who was a friend of Fothergill and had lived at Burtersett a few miles away. Hillary, also a Quaker, had gone even farther afield than Fothergill and published his best known book on the climate and epidemics in Barbados, where he was physician for ten years. Will and his young medical friend, Dr. (now Professor) Christopher Booth, also from Wensleydale and referred to above, have filled in a gap in medical history with an account of Hillary and his work.[37]

In September Will was presented at the Aysgarth Institute with a bound book containing the names of nearly all his patients in the dale, and a cheque, in recognition of his long and devoted service to the dales people. The inscription read:

"To Dr. W. N. Pickles, C.B.E. from his patients and friends, as a mark of the affection and esteem in which he is held, this book is presented as a token of friendship and gratitude for his fifty years service in the Dale."

The presentation was made by a lady who was the second baby introduced to the world by Will after his arrival in the dale fifty years earlier. The first had left the dale and could not be traced.

In his reply Will said:

"I arrived at Aysgarth Station by an early train on the 12th August 1912. I was met at the Station by the late Matt Sayer and driven to the village in a high dogcart.

"I had at that time not the slightest inkling that I was to spend more than a few weeks here, let alone the half century I have just completed. Yet within a very few days, it seemed extremely likely that I should join my old friend and fellow-student, Dean Dunbar, in this old-established practice.

"Thinking back, I cannot describe adequately the delight that I experienced right from the beginning of my life here. I had quite definitely fallen on my feet in what I might describe as the practice of my dreams.

"At Aysgarth I had congenial surroundings – to this day I have never lost the thrill of our beautiful dale; a congenial partner – never did man have a better partner than I had in Dr. Dunbar; but, as much as these, kindly cooperative patients, who were not slow to tell me how attached they were to their old doctors, but who were ready to give me a trial . . .

"I do thank you, my very dear friends of Wensleydale, for helping to make my life here so happy and I can only say that I would not have spent my life elsewhere for all the wealth of the Indies."

Not quite so many visitors from over the seas visited Aysgarth that year but old friends continued to drop in on a Sunday afternoon and often brought a visitor with them.

He continued to do a round every day, but his partner, who made out the visiting list, gave him less to do. The charts of infectious disease were still being maintained by Gerty from Will's notes, but it was difficult to obtain details of all the cases, as Will's share of the practice was now so much diminished.

In February 1963 he had a telephone call from Dr. Stephen Anning to ask if he would accept the Fellowship of the Royal College of Physicians of London. There is a substantial fee to be paid by the recipient of the F.R.C.P., and the concurrence of the person concerned must be obtained. For more than twenty years distinguished Fellows, including Professor Major Greenwood, Sir Edward Mellanby, Sir Wilson Jameson and Sir Ernest Rock Carling had been proposing Will's name, but his election had been opposed, because of a bye-law of the College which excluded any doctor in partnership. This virtually excluded general practitioners from the Fellowship because even if they were not at the time in partnership they might enter a partnership later. The wording of the bye-law was eventually changed so that a general practitioner in partnership

could, with special permission from the Censors' Board, be elected
to the Fellowship. As a consequence, in 1963, Will became the first
practising G.P. to become a Fellow of the College. Starting with the
modest Licence of the Society of Apothecaries, the L.S.A., Will had
achieved what is regarded by some as the highest British medical
qualification that a physician can obtain.

On 27th May he "gave faith" to the College and was admitted to
the Fellowship. Two days later he went to the offices of the General
Medical Council to register the new qualification and there by
chance he met an old acquaintance who was about to be struck off
the register for some chicanery connected with the use of a diagnostic
box. As he came out of the building he found himself thinking of
"fortune's buffets and rewards" and reflecting that he had on the
whole been one to whom fortune had proved kind.

The arthritis of the knees he had suffered from during his second
trip to the U.S.A. was now returning and making it increasingly
difficult for him to get about. After Christmas he went into hospital
at Harrogate for treatment, and much to his disappointment 1964
started for him in a hospital bed. His disability had become so acute
however that he was quite thankful to feel that something was being
done, particularly as he was under the care of a physician, Dr. T. G.
Reah, who was an old friend. Physical therapy and some weight
reduction brought about a rapid improvement, and within six
weeks he was able to return to Aysgarth again.

The winter dragged on. "No one comes to see us in this weather
so we are rather dull," he wrote.

That May he fell in the porch of his house and sustained a crush
fracture of one of the lumbar vertebrae. He again attended the Royal
Bath Hospital, Harrogate, for an X-ray examination and for some
more physiotherapy.

"I have scoffed at physiotherapy and all that mumbo-jumbo all
my life," he said later, "but when I needed it myself I found it did
a great deal of good."

In spite of this set-back he was soon getting about again, but he
felt that the time had come for him to retire finally and completely
from general medical practice.

And so in October 1964, he retired, six months before his eightieth birthday. Before he did so he went round the practice telling his old patients that the time had come for him to give up, recalling perhaps the words he had written many years before:

"It is unthinkable for us to change our habitat and we retire with reluctance, dreading that utter loneliness which would result from a separation from our work and from our patients."

His eightieth birthday, in March 1965, was marked by notices in many newspapers and medical journals.

The Practitioner, under the heading "G.O.M. of General Practice", referred to him as follows:

"On March 6, Dr. William Pickles, the grand old man of general practice, will celebrate his 80th birthday. Pickles of Wensleydale – as he will undoubtedly be known to future generations – has established for himself a niche in the history of medicine, of which England will be forever proud."

The Medical News reported an interview with him which included the following passage:

D.C.:   For a number of reasons there is much apathy – almost despair – amongst G.P.s today. Can you offer any advice for improving the situation?

W.P.:   I know what you mean and cannot suggest much for some of the causes. But I think that some G.P.s might be happier if they thought more of their opportunities.

D.C.:   Are there any?

W.P.:   Well, I meant from the point of view of studying mankind. Each one of us has the chance of adding a little to the sum of human knowledge, and most G.P.s consider that this would be nonsense. But nothing is farther from the truth. Our observations are direct and the contact is human and we can often supply facts which no other members of the profession can. We see disease in its early stages – very rarely a chance of a specialist – we can follow it through from the beginning to the end of the illness.

D.C.: Would this be true of a practice in an industrial area such as, say, Bolton?

W.P.: I think it would. Having many more patients to attend to, they would see many more aspects of disease.

D.C.: What is your attitude to G.P.s having higher degrees – do you think they are better doctors for them?

W.P.: I don't think the letters count. What is important is working for degrees and diplomas because it keeps you active and up-to-date.

D.C.: One final question. Is there anything you regret in your long and distinguished career?

W.P.: Only that I took up my epidemiological studies so late. Ten years earlier and I might have made some useful contributions.

Some of the non-medical press seized on the sentimental appeal of the occasion. "Dr. Cameron of the Dales says good-bye" was a typical headline. The B.B.C. wished to interview him but he declined.

In August Lord Woolton, who was staying in the neighbourhood, called on him. He had previously given Will a copy of his Memoirs in which he had written:

"I am honoured by the acceptance of this book by Dr. William Pickles who has helped so many people for so long, and who has done so much in the interests of Preventive Medicine."

By a strange coincidence Lord Woolton had been an assistant master in a school in Burnley when Gerty was a girl, and they were amused to discover that Gerty's parents used to entertain the head-master of this school whom, Gerty recalled, she and her sisters "hated with a deadly hate", a feeling which had apparently been wholeheartedly shared by the assistant master.

Visitors from other countries still came to see Will, including Dr. Popovic from Belgrade in 1964, and Dr. Bolotovsky, an epidemiologist from Moscow, in 1965. The latter turned to the British professor of microbiology who had accompanied him and referring to Will's charts said rather bluntly, "this is the sort of medicine you should be doing".

Time passed more slowly now. They acquired a television for the first time so that Will could watch the cricket, and he continued to read a lot. He had lost three stone since his admission to hospital in 1964, his arthritis was much better and he could walk up to one mile each day. One night in July 1965 he experienced a pain in the right calf and his foot went cold and numb due to a partial occlusion of his posterior tibial artery. Two days later he was admitted to Scotton Banks hospital in Knaresborough and from there was transferred to the Royal Bath hospital in Harrogate. Nothing was done except that he was given, as he said, two effective vaso-dilators, nicotinic acid and whisky.

Perhaps they did not think too well of his chances in hospital as one day a parson arrived and offered to pray with him. Will politely declined. "I would have felt such a hypocrite," he said afterwards. "I really cannot believe in a good God. Look at all these wars that are going on. Nature really is red in tooth and claw." He seemed to be reconciled to partial invalidism after he returned home at the end of August and when I saw him early in September that year he was not dressing each day but pottering about in the bungalow in his dressing-gown. He was as cheerful and sanguine as ever and again said, "I have had a happy life. I have been very lucky."

In September he was re-admitted to hospital and at the end of the month the right leg was amputated below the knee. "I never had a moment's anxiety," Will said afterwards. "I never thought about it". Unfortunately the wound did not heal properly as the circulation was inadequate, and three weeks later a further amputation high up on the thigh had to be done. He had to have a blood transfusion and when the surgeon came round the next morning and asked him how he was, he replied, "I'm feeling very well indeed. It must be the two pints of young Christian blood you pumped into me."

He had a few 'phantom' limb pains, but "nothing that would make me shout out".

Hardly a day passed while he was in hospital without a visitor, including "all the clergy of the neighbourhood and the Bishop of Ripon".

One letter from Askrigg pleased him greatly:

Dear Dr. Pickles,

All we village people are so relieved to hear that your operation is over and your condition is satisfactory.

Rose McClurg and myself have been round the village calling on all asking them to attach their signatures on the accompanying "Get Well" card for you.

It would indeed have warmed your heart to hear the expressions of genuine concern for your welfare and the great love and affection all have for you . . . it has absolutely amazed me when going round how much you mean to all the villagers. They often recalled a special word or incident in connection with one of your visits. Your interest in their families – remembering their births and always asking sympathetically about their children's future.

The card is perhaps a bit worn-looking but it has been in so many hands . . .

Our love to you.

Dot Outhwaite

There followed 179 signatures, some in the tremulous handwriting of old age, and after others the names of all the children, "and Tom and Isabel" . . . "and Harry, Nora, Esther and Allan".

He came home on the 18th November, a cold misty day, and the only time he felt at all sorry for himself was when the ambulance made a long detour to deliver or pick up patients in the surrounding country. They made calls at Bedale, Catterick, Richmond and Preston-under-Scar before at last bringing him home. The much loved district nurse, Nurse Abraham, looked after him and taught him to be independent again. He soon managed to push himself round the bungalow in his wheel-chair and when a friend visited him he said in reply to a solicitous enquiry, "I've never been so happy before. I'm exulting in this new lease of life."

He continued to write recollections and stories about his pre-decessors for the "In England now" column of the Lancet, and occasional obituary notices of old friends. Of Dr. Hansell,[44] who had practised in Bedale with Dr. Eddison since 1914, he wrote, "His was one of those quiet lives with no fraction of self advertisement or flamboyance."

In April 1966 he was invited to be the guest of honour at the B.M.A. Teeside branch annual dinner at Catterick Bridge. David Shepherd, now the garage proprietor, called for him and Gerty, helped him into the car, folded up the chair and packed it in the boot and drove them to the hotel at Catterick Bridge. He was wheeled to the table where he took his place among the ninety-five guests. It was a time of intense, and sometimes bitter, negotiations between the B.M.A. and the Ministry of Health on remuneration and new conditions for G.P.s. Characteristically he started his speech by saying, "I am sick to death of medical politics and I expect you are too." So he spoke of the medical history of the dale and told them stories about his predecessors, Willis, Baker and Hime.

The Secretary of the branch, Dr. L. J. Rosin, in his letter of thanks wrote:

"It would be entirely superfluous for me to comment on the enjoyment derived from your talk by your audience.

"In your case it was abundantly clear that the Prophet is both respected and loved in his native land.

"The volume and spontaneity of the applause which followed your speech speaks more eloquently than any words I could possibly find to use."

In June they received a visit from Dr. William Dodd, Medical Officer of Health for Nottingham, and his wife. They delighted Will by giving him Lord Moran's book on Winston Churchill. Moran had been publicly criticised for publishing much of what he had learned in the course of his professional relationship with Churchill. Will, however, felt that the subject was of such great public importance and interest that he was justified in publishing the book. Dr. Dodd had got Lord Moran to sign the book and after he had read it Will, who had met Lord Moran on several occasions, wrote to him expressing his appreciation of the book. In his reply Moran wrote:

"Thank you for your kind letter and for what you say about my book which gave me great pleasure. It took me twenty-five years off and on to write it and I felt quite lost when it was finished."

Wooden ramps were built up to the front door so that Will could propel himself out into the garden in his wheel chair or to a waiting car. On many mornings that summer his old friend Cecil Riggs, who had been the village postmaster and who in semi-retirement still acted as part-time postman, called for him and took him on his rounds to Thornton Rust, Cubeck and Worton, and Will's old patients came out on to the road to talk to him again.

He had always read a lot, about two books a week, and now he began to re-read the books he had enjoyed in years long past: Dickens and "Ivanhoe", Arthur Bryant's history, Gibbon's *Decline and Fall*, and the Old Testament. He watched a lot of cricket on television. "I think I like watching cricket more than anything else in the world," he said – a feeling not shared by Gerty.

At the beginning of 1967 he had a severe pain in the chest. "I could only diagnose it as pressure on the nerves very like secondaries in the spine," he wrote. "It was obviously not that as I am quite free now." The probability that the pain was due to a small cardiac infarct does not seem to have occurred to him.

In May the College of General Practitioners became, by Royal Command, the Royal College of General Practitioners, an event which pleased Will immensely. General practice was beginning to achieve the high status which he had always believed it merited. A month later the College established a William Pickles lectureship, and Dr. P. S. Byrne, general practitioner and later director of the department of General Practice at Manchester University, was invited to deliver the first lecture which he did in 1968.

Towards the end of January 1969, I received a letter from Will:

"My prostate is playing me up and will give me a hell of a time soon, so my considered opinion is that it will have to go ... I know it's a risk but the certain alternative does not mean a long life or a pleasant one."

And so at eighty-three he faced with his usual equanimity what was probably at best a fifty-fifty chance of survival. He was admitted to hospital and the operation was successfully carried out on Monday, 24th February. He seemed to be making a good recovery but on Saturday of the same week he developed pneumonia. He was semi-conscious' the next day and did not recognise Gerty when she came. He died that night.

The funeral was held in Aysgarth Church on Thursday, 6th March. It was a cold, brilliant, sunny day. Some snow still lay along the dry stone walls and the grass was buff coloured from being covered for weeks with snow. It was the sort of day when you feel that winter must at last be over, and yet the signs of spring have not appeared.

The church was packed with Will's old patients who had come from up and down the dale. The Wensleydale G.P.s and old medical friends from far afield were there, and all who had known and loved him felt that their own world was diminished by his death.

The young clergyman who officiated at the service referred to Will's agnosticism, but assured his listeners that God chooses all sorts of people to do his work. Somehow I was reminded of the remark of Will's predecessor, Dr. Baker, when he said on his deathbed that he "only dealt with the Head of the firm".

On 23rd April a Memorial Service was held in the Church of Emmanuel at Leeds. The President of the Royal College of General Practitioners, Dr. John Hunt, and other members of the College Council were there, together with members of the Yorkshire faculty of the College, representatives of the University of Leeds and its medical faculty, and Will's G.P. friends.

The choir of his old school, Leeds Grammar School, sang an anthem by Byrd.

The record is finished. Will Pickles will remain in the memory of his friends as long as they live, but his work and the inspiration it has given to general practitioners all over the world, will, I believe, last as long as medicine itself.

20

RETROSPECT

GERTY SURVIVED WILL by only five months. Soon after his death she revealed that she had been feeling ill for some time, and after full investigation it was found that she had advanced cancer of the stomach. Perhaps she had concealed the symptoms in order to spare Will; certainly after his death she declined rapidly and died that summer in a Harrogate nursing home.

Soon after these sad events I drove up to Aysgarth for a last visit, and as I came into the dale my thoughts went back to the first locum I did for Will Pickles in July 1949.

I had been in low spirits at that time because of a family bereavement, but I remembered that as I had driven the last few miles from Wensley to Aysgarth through West Witton and Swinithwaite, the peace of this most English scene had seemed to permeate and soothe my mind.

Once again I looked over to the right where the square towers of Bolton Castle dominated the hills above Redmire, while on the left massive Penhill rose steeply to its high moor, and all between stretched lovely fertile Wensleydale. There was an occasional glimpse of the river Ure winding along the middle of the dale and I recalled again the sweet smell of the cut hay lying in the afternoon sun on that first visit.

I stayed at the George and Dragon that year and every year that I went back to Aysgarth. This was essential, as the "doctor's bed-room" at the inn had a private line to the antiquated little telephone exchange in the surgery which was also connected to Madge the dispenser's house, so that urgent enquiries could be made by the locum about important details such as, where exactly did the patient live, or on what shelf could the penicillin be found.

At that time the George and Dragon was kept by Harry Holmes, who was stone deaf. It was then an unpretentious country inn, facing sideways and jutting out on the corner at the entrance to the village. The next landlord, Bill Douglas who took over in 1953, with great energy carried out many improvements, but in the process the inn lost something of its purely village character.

In those earlier days the public bar was so small that when Harry Cockburn, Tom Percival and Willie 'Postie' had settled down for the evening, it seemed full. The Yorkshire wit and eloquent silences of these old dalesmen have now been largely replaced, in the summer at least, by the friendly chatter of week-end visitors from Bradford or Leeds, and the tankards of draught ale supplanted by gin-and-tonics.

Sometimes on a hot afternoon when there were no calls to be made I went for a swim in the river above the Aysgarth Falls. Each year I returned to these banks to watch the dippers and pied wagtails bobbing and darting by the rippling water and to think about the experiences which general practice brings. In a single morning the G.P. is indeed often confronted by the whole fate of man, from the kicking foetus within its mother's belly, to the miserable, decrepit old man waiting for death to release him. You suddenly come right up to a person, like the television camera when it moves in to focus on someone's face. You see their fears and how they are at grips with life.

The Aysgarth practice at that time was almost entirely based on consultations in the houses of patients, and it was not long before I became acquainted with the homes and lives of a good many of the three thousand or so patients. Each year that I returned I felt more familiar with these kindly people, and they grew used to seeing me. As one old man re-visited put it: "Aye you were the relief man. I remember."

I came to appreciate the very important and privileged position the G.P. can occupy in his community. Indeed quite often he plays a part in people's lives of which he is not even aware and may discover only by accident. His opinion may carry much more weight than he thinks and he should never brush off or laugh at his patients' confidences although sometimes he cannot fail to be astounded at the importance which may be attached to things which to him may seem trivial.

An elderly maiden lady said to me on the round one morning, "Have you got time to come and see my dog's grave doctor? I've made her a garden of remembrance". She was a London cockney of some wit transplanted to Wensleydale and at first I thought she was joking. I followed her out to the back garden, however, and there under an apple tree was a curved path made of stone flags and leading up to a mound of stones on which rock plants were flowering. "Nice ain't it", she said. "How d'you think she'd have liked that?" I realised then that the mongrel bitch which lay buried there had been very important in this lady's life.

If the round is not too rushed what a rich commentary it provides – material for a Maupassant or Tchechov. It is easy, particularly when hurrying back late for lunch, to be curt with a "difficult" patient. A middle-aged woman was disagreeable and impatient when I called and I was on the point of leaving her rather abruptly when a hideous girl of thirteen staggered into the room. She was a spastic and mentally defective. This was the woman's only child and she was also nursing an old man, a distant relative, who lay dying upstairs. She had some reason to feel dissatisfied with what life had brought her.

In a play the dialogue can be made to fit a tragic theme, but in ordinary life conversations are often quite incongruous. I find in my notes the record of a little conversation with an educated woman patient aged seventy-seven.

"My husband left me four years ago – Wait a moment, I've left the milk on . . . Oh the lies, doctor. You've no idea."

Such moments are not uncommon in a G.P.'s life. If he can give time to listen with sympathy, he can probably do more than a cataract of medicine to "cleanse the stuffed bosom of that perilous stuff that weighs upon the heart".

I used to visit the postman in one village year after year. He suffered with valvular heart disease and found it increasingly difficult to do his round, although he was only in his forties. One night he died suddenly in bed.

"He put his arms round me," said his wife, "and then drew his head back and said 'your hair tickles'. Then he died."

There are plenty of comedies too. I was called to an inn in a distant village late one evening. "A bit of a contretemps here tonight doctor," said the innkeeper with considerable sang-froid. "Will you go upstairs?"

As I climbed the narrow stairs I heard a baby's cry, and there of course was the young mother who had been sitting in the bar most of the evening until "the waters broke" just before closing time. A few minutes later the district nurse rushed in, and in the poor light she put her bag down on top of the unfortunate baby which I had placed in an armchair. Hearing it cry, she snatched the bag away and then tripped over the light cable, pulling it out of the socket, and plunging us all into darkness. The bedroom was in a fearful mess and in the confusion of closing time, with people singing and dogs barking, we couldn't even get the essentials for rural midwifery – brown paper and boiling water. However, the nurse remained calm, emptied a chest drawer to make a safe place for the baby, and started to clean up.

Sometimes if one is rushed the most important problem in a household may be missed. Talking to the niece of a robust old man of ninety, who was recovering from pneumonia, and feeling rather pleased with the result, I spoke enthusiastically about the wonders of penicillin and the vigour and vitality of this stout old man when I suddenly realised that the niece, an elderly lady who had been nursing the old man, now needed more attention than he did. She had been up with him for several nights while he had been rambling and trying to get out of bed. Now she was on the point of collapse with nervous exhaustion. Who teaches the medical students these things? Indeed is it possible to teach these aspects of medicine in the intensive but somewhat unnatural conditions of the hospital ward?

Old people take up more and more of the time of the G.P. today. But the young doctor may learn much from them. "What does it feel like to be eighty-four?" I asked one old lady who had nothing definitely wrong with her but who, because of her age, was on the monthly visiting list. "Well doctor", she replied with a slow drawl, "some days I fale eight-four and others I fale like a girl of eighteen."

A good many of these old people had out-lived their friends and had no relatives with whom they could live. When asked what was wrong they would sometimes say, "I think maybe I've lived too long doctor", or "It's time I was shifting. You stay till you're not wanted, doctor."

They sit in their little kitchens all day and the ivy grows slowly across the window-pane and then through the cracks and crevices into the house.

At the other end of the scale are the children who still take up a large proportion of the G.P.'s time.

During these locums it was a joy on a sunny morning to see the schoolchildren bursting out of the little primary school on to the green at Bainbridge, in their white shirts or red and blue cardigans – shouting and laughing or perhaps standing quite still and gazing gravely at something which had caught their attention. The children of Wensleydale are shy, but when they are used to you, friendly and informative. One four-year-old sitting on the wall gossiping with two other fair-haired little girls like sparrows called out to me as I got out of the car: "It's not me that's poorly it's Nan and I've had the measles."

Sometimes I would pause on the round at Yore Bridge grammar school and stand for a little while under the trees by the road to watch a cricket match between the older boys and girls. There was something eternal about the scene, an echo from ancient Greece perhaps – the boys all in white, leaping in the sun to catch a ball or making a graceful stroke, and the girls with brown legs flashing beneath their white skirts running swiftly across the field.

The scene was not always so happy. Bovine tuberculosis was not uncommon when I first went to the dale, and I remember trying to reassure one young farmer about the illness of his four-year-old boy, who was in hospital with glandular tuberculosis, probably contracted from the milk from his father's herd. In general, however, I found the children of the dales wonderfully healthy and their demeanour more grave and pleasing than that of the city children. They had plenty of fun. There were always two or three village fêtes, outings or sports days during the time I was there each year and at these there was quite a family atmosphere. Cousins raced against cousins, and fathers against uncles on the wide village greens of West Burton or Bainbridge. After one sports day there was an outbreak of vomiting and diarrhoea, derived, I suspect, from corned-beef sandwiches. From the epidemiological point of view it was fascinating to follow the infection as it spread like a heath fire through many of the families.

Fortunately, for the good of our souls, not all patients have a blind trust in doctors. One of the kindest and wisest men in the dale was Fred Lawson, the Yorkshire artist who lived very simply in a little house in Castle Bolton and who did not regard doctors as infallible. He went to Castle Bolton for a holiday in 1911 and stayed there until his death in 1968. He had therefore lived in the dale since the time of Dr. Hime, who preceded Will in the practice. He remembered Hime as "a smart young fellow who left his top hat and kid gloves on the kitchen table". His comments on the Aysgarth doctors and life in general were kind but pithy. Of Will he said:

"Will Pickles doesn't just come in and out saying 'We'll send a bottle of medicine along'. He stops and chats and gives confidence. That's what a lot of these old people want. You'd be surprised how much medicine ends up down the sink."

Of the summer visitors he said:

"People come up here expecting it to be like the railway posters. They fale chated if it's pouring with rain," and in a reflective vein he continued, "Why do they always show people lying down on the holiday posters? That's no good. Folk should do something different on holiday."

His comments on disease sometimes seemed to me to be very near the truth. I was discussing the frequency of coronary thrombosis with him one day when he remarked:

"All that sitting about in cars and then sitting down in the house is no good, it lets the stuff accumulate. It's like a house, if you don't shove the stuff around things begin to pile up in the corners."

He had chronic blepharitis and his vision was fading when I saw him last. He was still painting, however, and said, "I couldn't paint so well if my eyes were good – I'd see too much." Living and

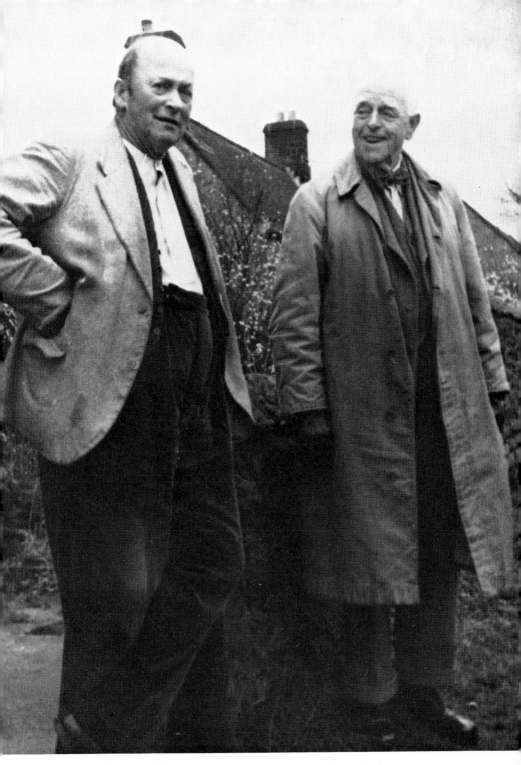

A roadside consultation: Fred Lawson and Will

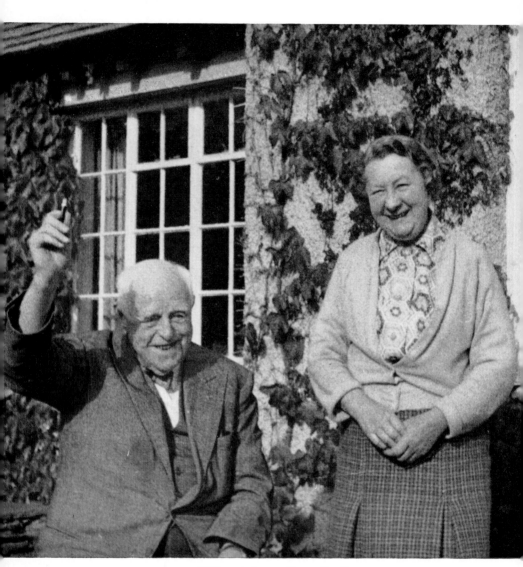

Will and Gerty: "Goodbye"

painting for half a century in the quiet peace of Castle Bolton had given him a wise philosophy:

"Why worry about all these rockets? They're not to be compared with the rocket that gets us all in the end."

"What's the use of hurrying, they've got the scale wrong, the whole thing is only as big as that" (pointing to the tip of his little finger).

"The vital part of life hasn't got any bigger, the journey was just as important when you went on a donkey."

Of the India–Pakistan war: "It's wasteful. It takes so long to make a man."

"It's all the ordinary people who don't understand politics who keep things swate."

Fred was once asked by the Wensleydale society to talk about painting at one of their meetings in the Institute.

"Well," he started off, "what can I tell you about painting – everyone has his own views on that. But I'll try and answer your questions though I don't know as I'll know all the answers," and he sat down.

But then, in the words of Madge, "He went yarning on so that it was the most enjoyable afternoon I have ever had."

Fred Lawson's water-colours vividly convey the seasons and the climate of the dale. He went painting in all weathers and was quite content to sit out behind his house in the snow painting the silent winter scene with the sun glinting on the side of a footprint, and the grey mass of Penhill rising from the mist in the background.* His pictures, and those of other Yorkshire artists such as George Graham and George Jackson, are to be found in all types of houses in the dale, from the big house to the tiny cottage. It is said that the village tradesmen were sometimes paid in water-colours by these Wensleydale artists when they were short of money, and if this is true they were well paid.

I was always delighted to find their water-colours in the sitting

* Fred Lawson died towards the end of 1968. The large retrospective exhibition of his paintings held in Middlesborough Art Gallery in 1969 confirmed the great talent as a water-colour painter possessed by this simple and profound man.

o

rooms of the little shops, hanging beside a wedding photograph perhaps showing the patient as the mustachioed groom and soldier in the 1914–18 war, and alongside that another more faded photograph of grandfather playing ring-a-ring-a-roses with white pinafored little girls, now grandmothers themselves. The sense of the continuity of life in an English village is very strong.

The general practitioner has a more intimate relationship with the dying than the hospital doctor. He has often known them for years, and perhaps has to care for them over a long period in their last illness. The arguments for euthanasia may often appear powerful to him. An old man dying from an incurable disease said, "One ought to be given something rayther to sleep one away."

The district nurse plays a most important part in the country. Sometimes she is also the midwife, school nurse and health visitor as well, and she knows her people intimately. She is with the mothers during childbirth, she is often the first on the scene when an accident in the home or field occurs, and she is the daily or twice daily visitor of the dying. Many, like nurse Abraham at Askrigg, come to be greatly loved and trusted by their people. On one occasion this nurse curtailed her summer holiday to come back and keep an eye on a patient she was nursing through a long illness, because she thought the relief nurse from a distant village might not "understand" her patient. The country doctor recognises the nurse's car from afar, and often draws up alongside to get the latest information about a patient and to give some fresh instructions.

The material conditions of the lives of the people of Wensleydale have changed a lot since I first went to Aysgarth twenty years ago. The four passenger trains in each direction that used to wind their way through the dale and were used by Will and his partners in the early days to take acutely ill patients to hospital, no longer run. First the passenger service closed down, then the goods service, and now they have taken up the rails.

Instead of the trains the village people use the buses, but even these are beginning to be less used as more and more families have cars or friends who will give them a lift to the town or the doctor's surgery when required.

Each year I went back to Aysgarth I noticed that the farms were better equipped not only with machinery outside but also inside. Refrigerators and washing machines appeared, the old stone flags were covered with bright linoleum or Marley tiles and the flower-patterned wallpaper was replaced by paper with modern abstract designs. When I remarked to one mother that the forest of TV aerials had rather spoiled the appearance of one of the most beautiful villages she replied rather sharply, "I don't think it's too many. We have no cinemas or theatres you know."

The "P.A.I." (public assistance institution) at Bainbridge, now the local authority home for the elderly, improved enormously under successive "masters" and more humane legislation. When I first went to see patients there the smell and appearance of the workhouse still prevailed, the old men sat idly and silent in one part of the building and the old women in another. Later on, the cold stone floors were covered with cork tiling and carpets, and electric radiators were installed on the bathroom walls. Each man had his own Harris tweed suit, there was TV in the sitting-room, individual sewing lockers for the women, and both sexes sat down together for meals at tables for four in the dining room.

Other changes were taking place as in many other country areas of England. Working horses have disappeared from the farms and the introduction of complex agricultural machinery has meant that there are fewer jobs for men and women. The colourful visiting Irishmen who used to come to help get the harvest in are no longer required.

Young men and women, especially the more intelligent, now go off to Darlington, Leeds or London to work, and in their place come retired couples from these and other cities; couples who had perhaps when younger enjoyed their summer holidays in the dale. Now they are buying up the cottages and putting in central heating and other improvements the previous tenants had never known. The increasing proportion of elderly people has meant more work for the doctors, and only too often one of an old couple has died soon after retirement, leaving the survivor to live on alone.

When Will went to Aysgarth in 1911, the population of Aysgarth Rural District was 4,262, by 1961 it had declined to 3,303 and the proportion of old people, particularly old women, had increased.

In spite of all the changes which have taken place in the rural areas, the country doctor still has a uniquely important part to play and his life remains one which can be full of interest and satisfaction.

General practitioners in the cities are sometimes criticised as being "mere form fillers and signposts", and others are said to feel frustrated because they think that if they do not accede to every whim of their patients that the patients will leave them for a more "amenable" doctor. I think this depressing picture of the city practitioner has been greatly exaggerated and in the country it is certainly not true. He may be the only doctor over quite a large area. His patients are usually loyal to him, and if he is any good at all a rewarding bond of friendship and trust develops between them. Such was certainly the experience of Will Pickles. As he himself said in concluding his Cutter lecture at Harvard in 1948:

"I do hope I have been able to pass on to you a little of the atmosphere of a busy country practice in England, and as I speak from thirty-seven years personal experience, it is a full and happy life. It may, of course, be a mere repetition of irksome tasks, but this is probably the fault of the practitioner who, like Bunyan's man with the muck-rake, rakes to himself the straws and sticks and dust of the floor and can look no way but downward regardless of the crown which is being held above his head."

APPENDIX 1

PUBLISHED WORKS BY DR. W. N. PICKLES

1	Vincent's Disease	1919	J. Roy. Nav. Med. Serv. *5*, 87
2	Epidemic catarrhal jaundice: an outbreak in Yorkshire	1930	Brit. med. J. *1*, 944
3	Sonne dysentery in a Yorkshire dale	1932	Lancet *2*, 31
4	"Bornholm" disease: account of a Yorkshire outbreak	1933	Brit. med. J. *2*, 1178
5	Epidemiological opportunities of a country practice	1934	Univ. Leeds Med. Soc. Mag. *4*, 17
6	Epidemiology in country practice	1935	Proc. Roy. Soc. Med. *28*, 37
7	Epidemic catarrhal jaundice: with special reference to its epidemiology	1936	Brit. J. Ch. Dis. *33*, 192
8	Epidemic myalgia in children	1937	Brit. J. Ch. Dis. *34*, 85
9	Epidemic catarrhal jaundice	1939	Lancet *1*, 893
10	*Epidemiology in Country Practice* (with a preface by Prof. Major Greenwood)	1939	John Wright, Bristol. Re-issued 1949
11	Epidemic disease in English village life in peace and war. (An abridgement of the Milroy lectures for 1942)	1942	Univ. of Leeds Med. Mag. *12*, 64
12	*Control of common fevers*, Ed. R. Cruickshank. Chap. on "Catarrhal Jaundice"	1942	Lancet, London
13	A rheumatic family	1943	Lancet *2*, 241
14	The country doctor and public health	1944	Public Health *58*, 2
15	Epidemic nausea and vomiting	1944	The Medical Annual 109
16	John Jagger Pickles. Obituary	1944	Brit. med. J. *2*, 604
17	Harold Dobson Pickles. Obituary	1945	Brit. med. J. *1*, 64
18	Epidemic respiratory infection in a rural population with special reference to the influenza epidemics of 1933, 1936–7 and 1943–4	1947	J. of Hyg. *45*, 469 (with Burnet, F. M. and McArthur, N.
19	The country doctor	1948	Lancet, *1*, 201
20	Research in general practice	1948	Brit. med. J. *2*, 469
21	Epidemiology in country practice (The Cutter lecture delivered at the Harvard School of Public Health, Boston, Mass. April 12th 1948)	1948	New Eng. J. Med. *239*, 419
22	Chapter on "Infectious Diseases and the Country Doctor"	1949	*Science News* No. 12 Penguin Books

23 A happy adventure   1949   Surgo. Glas. Univ. Med. J. *15*, 90
24 George Cockroft. Obituary   1949   Lancet *1*, 504
25 A general practitioner's reflections   1950   Health Bulletin Dept. Hlth. Scot. *8*, 32

26 Epidemiology in country practice   1951   Bull. Post Grad. Com. in Med. Univ Sydney *7*, 25

27 Research in general practice   1951   Bull. Post Grad. Com. in Med. Univ. Sydney *7*, 45

28 Trends of a general practice: a hun-   1951   The Practitioner *167*, 322
    dred years in a Yorkshire dale
29 Then and now   1953   Univ. Leeds Med. J. *2*, 103
30 And this was my path   1953   Univ. Leeds Rev. III, *4*, 1
31 Reginald Lawrence. Obituary   1954   Brit. med. J.
32 J. J. Anning. Obituary   1954   Brit. med. J. *2*, 601
33 Sylvest's disease (Bornholm disease)   1954   New Eng. J. Med. *250*, 1033
34 Epidemiology in the Yorkshire dales   1955   The Practitioner *174*, 76
35 Epidemiologija u praksi seoskog   1956   Zagreb. Zastita Zdravlja
    lijecnika
36 The general practitioner and the   1957   Zodiac 4 No. 1
    laboratory
37 William Hillary, M.D. (1697–1763)   1957   Brit. med. J. *1*, 102 (with Booth, C. C.)

38 A happy alliance – Address to Asso-   1957   Aberdeen Students Journal
    ciation of Clinical Pathologists at
    Harrogate, April 9th, 1954
39 General practice in the country. Part   1957   The Queen's Med. Mag. J. Birm.
    of a symposium on careers in medicine   med. School *49*, 86
40 F. R. Eddison. Obituary   1959   Brit. med. J. *1*, 1479
41 John Fothergill – a great son of a   1962   New Eng. J. Med. *266*, 1164
    Yorkshire dale
42 "Epidemic Myalgia" in *Curiosities of*   1963   Gollancz, London
    Medicine. Ed. B. Roueche
43 Stories about his patients and prac-   Lancet Nov. 2, 1963; Feb. 1, 1964;
    tice. Anon in "In England Now"   Ap. 25, 1964; Nov. 21, 1964; Ap. 10, 1965

44 A. W. Hansell. Obituary   1966   Brit. med. J. Aug. 13, 1966

Tape Recordings

From time to time Will was asked to record messages to be played at meetings which he was unable to attend, such as the inauguration of the College of General Practitioners in Canada and the occasion of the first Royal College of General Practitioners William Pickles lecture delivered by Dr. P. S. Byrne in Manchester in May 1968. These and copies of all his available papers have been deposited at the Brotherton library of Leeds University.

Charts

The epidemiological charts maintained by Will with the help of Gerty from 1931–63 have been deposited at the London School of Hygiene.

APPENDIX 2

WILLIAM NORMAN PICKLES 1885–1969

Qualifications and Honours

1909	L.M.S.S.A.
1910	M.B., B.S. Lond.
1914–19	Surgeon R.N.V.R.
1918	M.D. Lond.
1939	M.R.C.P. Lond.
1942	Milroy Lecturer, Royal College of Physicians, London
1946	Stewart Prize, British Medical Association
1948	Cutter Lecturer, Harvard University
1950	Hon.D.Sc., Leeds
1950	Vice-President, Section of General Practice, Royal Society of Medicine
1953	First President of the College of General Practitioners 1953–1956
	Bisset Hawkins Medal, Royal College of Physicians
1955	Hon. F.R.C.P. Edin.
	James MacKenzie medal, Royal College of Physicians, Edinburgh
1957	C.B.E.
1963	F.R.C.P. Lond.
1965	Hon. Fellow Royal Society of Medicine
	Hon. Vice-President British Medical Association

INDEX